Praise for
Grow Create Inspire

In *Grow Create Inspire*, Crystal Stevens has skillfully tied the
seemingly mundane—how to grow food, cook, shop, stay healthy—to
our deepest spiritual and transformative aspirations. In clear and often
poetic language, she chronicles her own journey toward a more self-reliant
yet deeply interconnected life, and makes this story useful to all of us by
sharing the recipes, techniques, and lessons she has learned or created
along the way. For anyone interested in homesteading, skill building,
and creating community, this book is an inspirational roadmap from
a guide who has blazed her own path toward sustainability.

—Toby Hemenway, author, *Gaia's Garden:
A Guide to Home-Scale Permaculture* and *The Permaculture City*

The perfect read for anyone searching to transform their time
on this earth into a truly satisfying journey! Crystal Stevens' passion for
the natural order shimmers throughout the text to energize and inspire,
while her knowledge and experience encapsulate the whys and how-to's
in the form of lists and anecdotal examples. Certainly a powerful
antidote for these times of decadent destruction -- full of wise words
and useful suggestions to help recreate Eden here on Earth.

—Jenni Blackmore, author,
Permaculture for the Rest of Us and *The Food Lover's Garden*

Grow Create Inspire embodies the hopeful, do-it-yourself attitude that
Mother Earth News has encouraged for more than 40 years. We're honored
that Crystal has found inspiration in our publication and has transformed
our ideals into a free-spirited, accessible plan for improving the health
of the Earth, our communities, and our own bodies and souls.

—Hannah Kincaid, Senior Editor, *Mother Earth News*

A healthy relationship between human society and the natural world
begins with a healthy relationship between individual humans and the
natural world. Crystal Stevens's *Grow Create Inspire* is as good a guide to understanding the building books of that relationship as you are going to find.

—H. Emerson Blake, Orion

Grow Create Inspire reads like a friendly chat with a dear friend
who is full of sage advice, shares fascinating experiences,
and has lots of great recipes to share.
—Deborah Niemann, author, *Homegrown and Handmade*
and *Raising Goats Naturally*

Grow Create Inspire is an excellent reminder and guide for
the importance of being connected to our food and ultimately
the earth. She simplifies the power of our consumption
and the important link to earth stewardship through
outlining clear goals any household can achieve.
—Dr. Julia Stevens, Microbial Ecologist,
North Carolina Museum of Natural Sciences

Crystal Stevens's lush and lyrical style make you feel like you're
hanging out with her around her homestead kitchen table, a one-on-one
lesson with an expert in sustainability. With step-by-step personal guidance
wrapped in empowering inspiration, this book makes sustainability
accessible while celebrating the beauty and creativity along the way.
—Lisa Kivirist, author, *Soil Sisters: A Toolkit for Women Farmers*
and *Homemade for Sale*

grow

create

inspire

crafting a joyful life of
beauty and abundance

∴ Crystal Stevens ∴

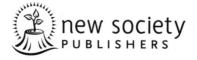

new society
PUBLISHERS

Cover design by Diane McIntosh.
Cover art: Woodblock print by Eric Stevens. Honeycomb art: © AdobeStock_65668768
Printed in Canada. First printing August 2016.

This book is intended to be educational and informative. It is not intended to serve as a guide. The author and publisher disclaim all responsibility for any liability, loss or risk that may be associated with the application of any of the contents of this book.

Paperback ISBN: 978-0-86571-837-1
EISBN 978-1-55092-632-3

Inquiries regarding requests to reprint all or part of *Grow Create Inspire* should be addressed to New Society Publishers at the address below. To order directly from the publishers, please call toll-free (North America) 1-800-567-6772, or order online at www.newsociety.com.

Any other inquiries can be directed by mail to:
New Society Publishers
P.O. Box 189, Gabriola Island, BC V0R 1X0, Canada
(250) 247-9737

LIBRARY AND ARCHIVES CANADA CATALOGUING IN PUBLICATION

Stevens, Crystal J., author
Grow, create, inspire : crafting a joyful life of beauty and abundance
/ Crystal Stevens.

Includes index.
Issued in print and electronic formats.
ISBN 978-0-86571-837-1 (paperback).--ISBN 978-1-55092-632-3 (ebook)

1. Permaculture. 2. Food crops. 3. Vegetable gardening. 4. Functional
foods. 5. Natural products. 6. Well-being. 7. Sustainable living. I. Title.

S494.5.P47S74 2016   631.5'8   C2016-904616-8
                                              C2016-904617-6

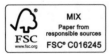 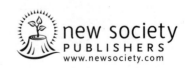

Funded by the Government of Canada | Financé par le gouvernement du Canada | Canada

New Society Publishers' mission is to publish books that contribute in fundamental ways to building an ecologically sustainable and just society, and to do so with the least possible impact on the environment, in a manner that models this vision.

MIX
Paper from responsible sources
FSC
www.fsc.org   FSC® C016245

Certified
B Corporation

new society
PUBLISHERS
www.newsociety.com

In loving memory of Carl V. Moore

Contents

Foreword

C RYSTAL STEVENS is an amazing renaissance woman. Not only is she my favorite farmer, she is a master herbalist, fantastic mother and artist. I met Crystal back when she was working at the Juice Bar at the local organic grocer in 2000. At that time I was in the thick of motherhood, bringing four children to the store all under the age of 7. I had just taken a break from my life as a busy pediatrician and was submersing myself in motherhood and sustainable living. By complete luck or destiny Crystal and I's paths have continued to weave together. My husband, also a physician, and I and the four kids all moved to a 100 acre farm in 2003 where we now can be even more sustainable with a large garden, orchard, chickens, honeybees and dairy goats for cheese making. Not long after that Crystal and Eric also moved to the farm they managed. Great minds think alike.

I admire Crystal's intelligence, curiosity and creativeness. Her latest creative act is the birth of a book that can change your life: Grow Create Inspire. Despite my broad understanding of the topics in this book, I still learned new things and was inspired to make further changes in my life to improve the world and brainstorm solutions to help heal the Earth. This book will teach you the importance and fundamentals of gardening at any level.

These pages will teach you how to heal not only your self with food and herbs but to do so while also healing Mother Earth. There are charts to determine which weeds you can use for health and nourishment from your yard and recipes to brighten your day. Crystal gives you the 'dirt' on how to grow your own veggies or mushrooms. There are stories that will inspire you to 'be the change you want to see in the world'. You will also get ideas on how to make Ecofriendly household cleaners, herbal lotions, and how to make a gift for a friend from recycled items. I recommend this book to you, a friend and every human on our precious planet! This book will become a well-worn friend and a perfect resource.

— Carrie Magill, MD
Integrative and Wholistic Physician, Mother, Organic Gardener

Preface

A FTER A DECADE AND A HALF of learning about healthy living, environmental stewardship and growing food and medicine, I have condensed my experiences into a book that is somewhat of a how-to guide for those beginning their adventures in eco-living and gardening. It can be a friendly reminder to those who are already incorporating eco-principles into their lives, a breath of fresh air to those who have dedicated their lives to the cause (knowing that younger generations are doing their part) and a guidebook for those just starting out.

Some material in this book has been taken from previously published works of mine, including *Permaculture, GRIT, Feast, The Healthy Planet, Mother Earth News, Mother Earth News* blog and my own *Grow Create Inspire* blog.

Gratitude

T HIS BOOK IS DEDICATED TO MY LOVING FATHER, CARL V. MOORE, from whom I inherited my love for nature and the great outdoors, the spirit of adventure, a strong work ethic, endless ambition and his giant stack of *Mother Earth News* magazines. I miss you ... something fierce.

To my mother, Cathy Moore, who continues to encourage and support me in all of my endeavors. Thank you for all of the hug-a-bunch sessions as a child and for making me feel like I could do anything I put my mind to. Thank you for teaching me the self-lessness and strength it takes to be a mother.

To my sister, Candice Moore, for always believing in me, for our uplifting conversations and for always making me laugh so hard that it hurts.

To my brother, Jason Crawford, for being a pillar of strength in our lives and for giving me loving support and encouragement.

To my husband, Eric Stevens ... Thank you for your infinite love, patience, support and encouragement. Your altruistic spirit and desire to make the world a better place inspires me greatly. To your parents, Ann and Barry, for their wonderful support

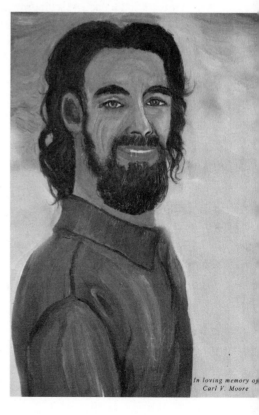

*In loving memory of
Carl V. Moore*

throughout the years and for raising such an amazing, thoughtful, creative, and loving son.

> Love must be as much a light as a flame.
>
> — Henry David Thoreau

To my children: I am honored and full of gratitude to be your mother. You bring joy and inspiration to my heart. Cay, you are a miracle. Your awe and wonder bring joy to me daily. Your talent astounds me. You are a magician with the pencil. Your inherent loving kindness leaves me hopeful for the future. You are wonderful. I love you. Iris, your brilliance amazes me. The love you have for nature makes my heart sing. You are such a wonderful helper in the garden and the kitchen. You are beautiful, my darling. Never stop filling your acorn pockets. I love you.

To all my dearest friends, mentors, teachers and family members ... You have all left huge impressions throughout my years. You have inspired my endeavors and helped to sculpt my path. I have an endless well of gratitude, love, respect and admiration for your role in helping me to navigate my way.

Introduction

G ROW CREATE INSPIRE is a practical guide for becoming more aware and more self-sufficient in all aspects of life, from physical health to mental well-being, relationships to self-confidence, reflection to goal-setting and so much more. This book is meant for all those multitalented beautiful minds and free spirits, all the thinkers, dreamers, artists, musicians, writers, poets, philosophers, educators, gardeners, farmers and anyone who ever wanted to leave a legacy on this Earth. Most of us are born with the amazing gift of an intrinsic moral obligation to the Earth, but sadly for many, it is lost throughout the maze of life. The speed at which our society moves is frightening. In less than a century, we have advanced so far in technology that looking into each other's eyes has become a lost art. We find it so hard to have a simple conversation without the casual mention of Facebook, Twitter, Instagram or Pinterest. We expect an instant response to electronic communication. Our brains have been wired to function so fast that it is virtually impossible to relax and meditate in silent thought without conscious, dedicated practice. Our Earth is being destroyed while we are too distracted to notice or too overwhelmed by our hectic lives to begin the work of Earth-healing. We find comfort in humor and mind-numbing entertainment. Children can recognize more corporate logos than they can vegetables or plants and trees in their own backyards. Yet children are some of the most curious and inspired individuals in our society. The philosophy of Grow Create Inspire focuses on the importance of allowing children to explore the Earth and to form a deep connection to our planet so that they will grow into the next generation of Earth stewards. My hope is that anyone who reads this book will be inspired to grow and learn, no matter their stage in life.

Emphasizing inspiration from the permaculture way of life, Grow Create Inspire touches on the various aspects of growth from personal growth

1

to growing your own food to growing for your future while leaving behind something more valuable than money for generations to come. In my lifelong search for individual solutions to environmental crises, words and phrases helped to describe my views but seemed not to express them fully throughout each aspect of my life. Sustainable, eco-conscious, eco-friendly, Earth steward, green, free-spirited, earthy — these were all good attempts at explaining the way I felt about the Earth, but I was still driving a car, buying gasoline, using paper and plastic and being a consumer. How could I label myself any of these if I was still consciously supporting the things I stood against? I was doing my part every day, I thought. I recycled everything possible; I wore hand-me-downs; I was a vegetarian; I was an activist; I grew food; I did river cleanups; I taught kids about environmental awareness; I rode my bike when I could. But I was still partaking in the very things that are depleting the Earth's natural resources. Even words like "green" and "sustainable" evolve into something other than their original meaning, and oftentimes their meanings are lost when exploited by major corporations trying to market their products.

My big ah-ha moments occurred within months of each other, right around my 18th birthday. Reading the book *Ishmael* by Daniel Quinn aloud with my father was one of those moments. The author's words painted a vast picture pinpointing the demise of civilization to the industrialized agrarian lifestyle. And it made so much sense to us. It was the moment when individuals, tribes, villages and cultures went from being self-sufficient hunters and gatherers tending the crops to being reliant on others for food. We hashed out the world's problems for hours that early morning in the springtime, covering everything from greed to war to hunger to politics to natural disasters and everything in between. The other ah-ha moment was when I first learned the term "permaculture." I was in a group called Eco-Act, founded and facilitated by the Missouri Botanical Garden in 1981 to inspire Earth stewardship in youth. My mother helped me sell chocolate bars so I could afford a trip to the Punta Mona Center for Sustainable Living and Education, an organic permaculture farm in Costa Rica.

In that day-long permaculture workshop, I felt fiery ambition running through my veins. It all became clear: permaculture could save the world! Well, at least it could if everyone in the world knew just how profound it was and if there were ways to simplify it to bring it to the masses in an accessible way. Permaculture became the one steadfast philosophy and way of life that I held dear to my heart throughout my 20s and 30s. Certified and specialized permaculturists all have different views on what it means to them and how to utilize it. That's the beauty of free will. And some permaculture experts may argue with my personal take on permaculture, but I do know this: it changed my life.

To me, permaculture is all-encompassing; it can be practiced every day in every single aspect of life in everything from thinking to dreaming, from building to restoring, from gardening to water conservation, from cooking to eating, from teaching to parenting and so much more. Permaculture is an umbrella under which all the innovative, resourceful Earth stewards may dream big while seeking shelter from the storms of this crazy world. Permaculture is inspiring. It stimulates the mind to think differently now for the future of the planet. Permaculture is alive with the possibilities of positive change.

As you read on, know that all suggestions are based on my experiences with the natural world, friends, family, mentors and the Earth itself, suggestions that can be adapted, altered and formatted to fit into your own life. Permaculture has sculpted my life and has opened many doors to my desire to deepen my connection to the Earth while implementing daily solutions to the problems facing the world today, and my hope in writing this book is to share this philosophy with others.

GROW | CREATE | INSPIRE

I watched the steam rise from my ceramic mug while envisioning a quest for my next creative endeavor. It was winter, one of those cold mornings where the stillness invites contemplation and intimacy. I was on the front porch, mesmerized by the reflection of the bare trees against the pale blue sky that was so vivid atop my coffee. The sun had just barely peeked over the horizon. I could see my breath. Our home is nestled in the forest. The sights and sounds of the forest in the winter made me ponder the rhythms of nature throughout the seasons. The plants were all dormant. Snow covered the rich dark earth, yet the forest was alive. Some of the trees had even begun to form buds despite the freezing temperatures. Nature, in all its glorious forms, is so resilient. I had an overwhelming sensation to grab my journal. The need to write took over every cell of my being. It was as though ignoring this feeling could literally cause a part of me to die inside. Ballpoint pen between my fingers, three words revealed themselves as I began to write: grow, create, inspire. Each word I followed with a loose interpretation or definition, as I understood them.

The dictionary sees it a little differently, of course, as definitions of these three poignant words are more literal than how I envision their true meaning.

To grow is to develop maturity. To create is to bring into existence. To inspire is to attribute influence. But when one truly grows, creates and inspires, our five senses manifest into something much greater than the mere sum of their parts.

Grow Create Inspire ...

Those three words written in my journal manifested into this book, which illustrates a holistic approach to healing the human spirit with environmental restoration as the ultimate goal. It focuses on mindfulness, compassion and resilience as tools for positive change. I hope this book will inspire individuals around the globe to discover a universal cure for Mother Earth's ailments. It discusses how the simple act of growing your own food can open the garden gates to welcoming the notion of a paradigm shift and inviting permaculture and other solution-based concepts in as a way of life. The goal of *Grow Create Inspire* is to encourage and empower others to do those three things — grow, create, inspire — on a physical and emotional level in every professional, personal and spiritual aspect of their lives. Brainstorming solutions for a healthier planet while thinking about ways to raise awareness and inspire mindfulness will bond a unified collective of Earth stewards. My hope is that *Grow Create Inspire* will resonate with everyone from all walks of life, especially in terms of carrying the torch of educating today's youth. In realizing that environmental issues are everyone's concern, we then begin to see the world through a clear lens. There are so many distractions pulling our attention away from the direction the world is headed in. *Grow Create Inspire* offers powerful solutions to some of the problems we face, all of which can be implemented by anyone around the globe with a little determination and support from their community. In the words of Margaret Mead, "Never doubt that a small group of thoughtful, committed people can change the world. Indeed, it is the only thing that ever has." To grasp a greater understanding of the interconnectedness of humans to one another, to nature and to the universe, and to discover what caused this massive disconnect with our Earth, is no new endeavor. Many of the great Earth stewards have pondered these thoughts, including Ralph Waldo Emerson, Henry David Thoreau, Mahatma Gandhi, Bill Mollison, Martin Luther King, Jr., Rachel Carson, Winona LaDuke, Vandana Shiva, Annie Leonard, Erin Brockovich, Chief Seattle and Ralph Nader. Continuing in the spirit of such great thinkers, *Grow Create Inspire* seeks to rekindle that fire within our hearts and renew our zeal for life in a way that allows us to form our own legacy of Earth stewardship and self-healing.

Grow Create Inspire focuses on the need for change in the way we grow food and addresses why the food crisis has become a global epidemic. The three sections (Grow, Create and Inspire) will discuss permaculture, growing food, reducing your carbon footprint, incorporating creative solutions into your personal life and making a direct impact in your own community by inspiring others to grow food and create positive change.

GROW will empower each of us to awaken our own personal growth by fostering a better future, one that can begin with the simple act of growing food in our own backyards. By truly grasping the basic concept of the vital importance of food for humans around the globe, we can begin to understand how to change the world, one small seedling at a time. Beyond the theoretical, this section will also cover basic gardening tips, permaculture projects and small-scale sustainable farming practices. The GROW portion also gives dozens of creative suggestions for encouraging friends, family and community members in this work. Community gardening, crop sharing, plant sales, seed swaps, guerilla gardening, workshops and sustainable backyard tours can bond and unite us in achieving these goals.

CREATE focuses on how we can create a world that works for everyone, and how we can collectively create a solution-based paradigm shift. This portion focuses on the importance of creativity to cultivating holistic sustainability and a world that is mindful, nurturing and compassionate — a world that is welcoming to everyone. Creativity is a vital component to human happiness and an essential ingredient to sustainability in its unadulterated definition. Through several examples of creativity in everyday life, whether it is cooking, food preservation, gardening, art, music, construction, writing or dancing, readers will see that they can easily adopt such activities into their life. CREATE includes recipes for happiness, stress release, healthy eating habits, holistic wellness and, of course, for homegrown, home-cooked meals and preserved foods.

INSPIRE acts as a cog for motivation. This aspect of the book includes uplifting and heartfelt stories of endurance, patience, excitement and inspiration. It also tells the brief stories of some of my own role models and how they have followed their dreams while doing their part for the Earth, inspiring thousands around the world. By acknowledging the lineage of your own inspiration, you can then begin to pay homage to Earth stewards who have taught you throughout your journey by sending ripples of positive change out into your own communities. It also shares stories of a few remarkable and innovative individuals who feel a sense of deep love for the Earth. These valiant folks brought their dreams of Earth stewardship to life and impacted millions along the way, changing the world as we know it. These individuals stand apart from the rest because they had undying ambition to make our world a better place.

Empowerment as a Solution to the Global Food Crisis

What if we empowered each other to plant the way for generations to come? What if we were able to bridge the gap between culture and cultivating — more specifically between cultural diversity and biodiversity — by simply having conversations with others? What if we were excited to hear and share stories of symbiotic relationships between people and people, plants and people, plants and the Earth: excited enough to make a difference in our own community? By illuminating the notion that real food (grown from the Earth) is the point at which all of these relationships intersect, we then begin to wrap our minds around the Earth as a living, breathing, holistic system that is in constant symbiosis. This holistic system is our home. Since the first humans walked upon the Earth, food has been a necessity for survival. The evolution of the importance of food to humans is remarkable. Food has sculpted civilizations. Food has been used to heal our bodies. Food defines us culturally. Food gives us pleasure. Food maps out the course of our everyday lives. For these reasons, food can change the future of the Earth.

Let us paint a beautiful oasis of food and abundance through backyard gardens, community gardens, sustainable farms and permaculture villages that purify our air, improve our water quality, give nutrients to the soil, provide nourishment to families and create habitats for pollinators. People from all walks of life are already uniting to form a global transition into an abundant, healthy, sustainable world and need a way to bring their dreams of this incredible future to fruition.

Grow Create Inspire reminds us of what already exists in our hearts and minds: how to be a conduit of change from within. Changes made within the self can ultimately inspire others, creating a ripple effect of concentric circles. As with any inspirational work, this book intends not to prescribe but to offer multiple approaches to sustainability. Readers can determine which solutions resonate most for them. A unified collective consciousness can be achieved if we inspire each other to, as Gandhi says, "be the change we wish to see in the world." I hope that you find *Grow Create Inspire* to be an altruistic, practical and meaningful approach to help make the world a better place.

grow

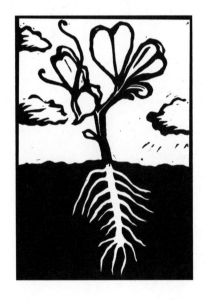

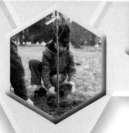

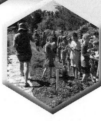
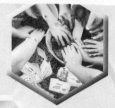
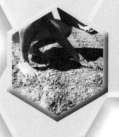

1

The Problems and the Solutions

Anything else you're interested in is not going to happen if you can't breathe the air and drink the water. Don't sit this one out. Do something. You are by accident of fate alive at an absolutely critical moment in the history of our planet.

— Carl Sagan

If we breathe air, drink water, eat food, enjoy sunshine, and cherish time to stroll through a park with our children and grandchildren, environmental issues affect us, each and EVERY ONE of us.

— Professor Pamela Garvey

U NLESS EACH OF US honestly acknowledges and assesses the negative impact we have on the Earth and actually puts solution-based thinking into practice, we cannot change the future of our home, planet Earth.

Understanding that the soil is a living, breathing organism covering the Earth, we then can implement simple solutions that everyone can take part in. It could be as simple as planting more trees or an organic garden with native pollinator-attracting plants. It could be as simple as removing a few items from your diet that contribute to soil degradation. It could be as simple as shopping locally or joining a CSA (community supported agriculture) farm. It could be as simple as taking public transportation. It could be as simple as buying less unnecessary stuff.

The soil is being destroyed at unprecedented rates by overconsumption, big business, human development, deforestation, monoculture, genetically modified foods, groundwater contamination, reliance on fossil fuels, unsustainable natural resource extraction and pesticide, herbicide and fungicide usage. All of these problems are symptoms of a deeper root cause: our massive disconnect from the Earth. The soil is the direct source of a significant amount of nutrients. We need the soil as much as we need the air, yet only a small percentage of people who care about these issues actually takes action to amend them. According to a survey conducted in 2013 by the Pew Research Center, 52 percent of Americans named protecting the environment a top priority for Congress, whereas 86 percent named strengthening the nation's economy as a top priority. Perhaps it's for those 86 percent that this quote was written: "Only after the last tree has been cut down. Only after the last river has been poisoned. Only after the last fish has been caught. Only then will you find that money cannot be eaten." (Cree Indian prophecy)

Anyone who has ever grown their own food or watched documentaries about food knows that this monoculture-based society not only is unsustainable, but is actually causing irreversible damage to the Earth every day. Despite this, we continue to support these practices, albeit sometimes unintentionally and out of convenience, whether buying prepared meals in unnecessary packaging or simply buying conventionally grown vegetables at the grocery store. Corn and soy are the crops with the most devastating contribution to monoculture. Unfortunately corn, soy and wheat are found in the majority of processed foods, especially in the United States.

Of course there are many practices that cause oftentimes irreversible soil degradation: fracking (hydraulic fracturing), oil drilling, mining, strip mining, deforestation and clear-cutting. Our reliance on fossil fuels is not helping. Unbeknownst to many, the simple acts of buying gasoline or using nonrenewable paper are also contributing to environmental degradation.

Access to environmentally friendly everyday products such as paper goods is very limited and often more expensive, making it impossible for those on a tight budget to choose to support the companies making a difference. And then there is air and water pollution. It is very hard to witness giant smokestacks lined up along major rivers that were clean and clear less than a century ago. I heard someone say over a decade ago that all of the oceans, rivers and streams are polluted beyond restoration. This news was devastating. How could humans, in less than 100 years, destroy the water supply around the world? How can we as a human race do our part to change the gloomy future of this planet? When an individual starts to brainstorm solutions, they seem practical and attainable considering the technology that is available.

For instance: what if big companies, factories and corporations simply stopped producing anything made from nonrenewable resources and instead made them from renewable resources such as agricultural waste, hemp and bamboo, and transitioned into powering their factories with renewable energy? Think of the positive impact that would make. Or on a larger scale — what if all the energy giants trained their current employees to operate energy plants using solar and wind power? What if all of the coal-fired and nuclear power plants simply converted to renewable energy? What if car companies were required by law to stop making gas-powered cars and only make hybrid or solar electric cars? The technology is available. There are many solutions to these problems.

However, each set of solutions has its own set of problems and unknown ramifications. So where does that leave us? When having this conversation with a dear friend and longtime environmental activist, Jim Scheff, his answer was, "We just need to use less." This is such a simple yet profound insight and is attainable with a little grunt work. Being an example to friends and family members in our own communities and sharing our stories big and small will send out ripples within our regions. There are plenty of individual solutions one could implement as well, which almost always have direct impact on others. The solution that I have adopted is food: how it can help heal our bodies and how it can help heal the Earth. Food is the basic necessity for survival. If everyone in the world knew how to grow their own food, that would reduce our reliance on large-scale industrialized agrarian production, ultimately reducing the need for fossil fuels, chemical applications and so much more. Food throughout communities would then become localized.

Problems Facing the World Today

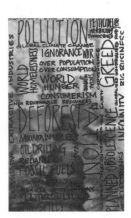

- Big Business
- Deforestation
- Globalized, industrialized food system
- Monoculture
- Mountaintop removal
- Pesticides, herbicides, fungicides
- Reliance on fossil fuels
- Exploitative extractive industries
- Oil drilling
- Oil spills
- Planned obsolescence of electronics and appliances
- Plastic culture
- Heavy metals
- Convenience

- Consumerism
- Reliance on electronics
- Overconsumption
- World hunger
- World homelessness
- War
- Massive disconnect to the Earth
- Greed
- Economic inequality

- Social inequality
- Social injustices
- Pollution
- Global warming
- Ignorance
- Prison injustice
- Medical-industrial complex
- Overuse of technology

Solutions for a Brighter Future

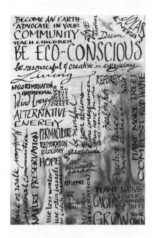

Be eco-conscious.

These are just a few solutions that you can implement in your home and community and see small changes:

- Plant more trees (they give us oxygen to breathe; they provide shelter for wildlife).
- Plant native flowers, shrubs and trees to attract pollinators and to create habitat for wildlife.
- Use alternative energy (solar, wind, hydro-electric, methane generation, geothermal, etc.).
- Grow a garden.
- Compost.
- Practice random acts of kindness.
- Reduce, reuse, recycle.
- Be resourceful and creative in everyday living.
- Be an advocate for the Earth.
- Become an activist in your community.
- Be holistic.
- Grow and make your own medicine.
- Create intentional communities.
- Bike or walk instead of drive when possible.
- Be mindful of your actions and their consequences.
- Use less water or use rain barrels.
- Make your own gifts.
- Practice peace.

- Try a little harder each day to make the world a better place.
- Find out how you can help protect the air, the water, the soil and the precious natural resources.
- Be an advocate for old-growth forests and the Earth as a living, breathing organism.
- Show a profound respect for the future of the Earth, which will inevitably inspire others to do the same.
- Work diligently to protect the environment for all those who inhabit the Earth and for future generations.
- Train coal and nuclear energy employees in alternative energy fields.
- Smile at a stranger.
- Practice compassion.
- Volunteer in your community.

What determines whether an individual does or does not become a steward of the Earth? Is it an intrinsic moral obligation? Is it a value taught to us by our families and communities? Are we born with an innate instinct to want to protect the Earth and its natural resources? How could anyone not care about the environment? Shouldn't it be the norm to want this world to be a better place? I've wondered about these questions for over a decade.

Some individuals seem to show no concern for the environment. How can we set positive examples for them and especially for children? Some individuals have more time, energy and resources to dedicate to ecological rehabilitation. But there are still solutions that everyone can implement, such as not littering and following the principles of the three R's: reduce, reuse, recycle. These don't take much effort at all.

For the future of the planet, our children need to grow up knowing how to be environmentally conscious, how to reduce their carbon footprint and how to encourage others to do the same. A quote by Chief Seattle, chief of the Duwamish tribe of the Seattle area, often comes to mind: "Teach your children what we have taught ours, that the Earth is our mother. Whatever befalls the Earth befalls the sons of the Earth. The Earth does not belong to man; man belongs to the Earth. Man did not weave the web of life; he is merely a strand in it. We do not inherit the Earth from our ancestors; we borrow it from our children." Whether or not we have children, the world as a whole has an obligation to pass Earth stewardship (possibly even as an ingrained character trait) down to the next generations. Some of the most profound wisdom comes from First Nations' chiefs. This wisdom alludes perfectly to the fact that sacred wisdom, and the wisdom passed on from generation to generation, cannot be broken even when the spirit is broken by an external force so vile. First Nations have been stripped of their basic human rights by the long process of colonialism, a project of land and human exploitation. Their land was ripped from under their feet, and while often ignored and forgotten today, the history and present, is absolutely heart-wrenching. They were on the land first, holding the land and all of its inhabitants with great reverence. They tried to live in harmony with the Earth; they treated the Earth with dignity. Because of their connection to the Earth and the seasons, the rhythms of nature, they held ancient wisdom in their hearts. This wisdom persisted despite the way they were treated by early settlers, despite the way they are treated by the government today. Reservations today are merely a fraction of what First Nations lived on.

There is a steadfast resistance of Native peoples to oppression with concern to indigenous land rights. There is indeed good and evil in the world, and as Woody Guthrie states, "some will rob you with a six gun and some with a fountain pen." The world is filled with naysayers and power-mongers. What European settlers did to the First Nations is sickening. In many ways, the project of colonialism lives on today in what scholars call neo-colonialism. Centuries of exploitation and persecution through slavery, colonialism and segregation created a deep scar in our society. I would call that scar racism. The racial separation and inequity in America is part of a thick barrier that has been building for centuries. It has taken an equal amount of time not only to regain trust but to regain dignity, and we as a nation are still working to dismantle these barriers. Kudos to all those who share the views of equality, who stand up for equal rights, who celebrate diversity and live with compassion and who are deeply hurt by the existence of racism. It is these individuals who have evolved past hatred, who have found light in the dark corners around the world, who have loved all life deeply and unconditionally. First Nations are a beautiful example of personal evolution and spiritual growth: holding so tight to virtuous love and compassion while suffering through the absolute hell that is genocide.

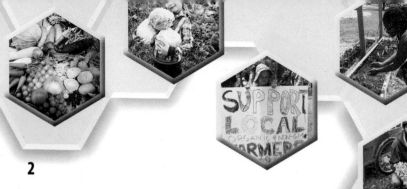

2

Food: The Common Thread that Weaves Humanity Together. Eat Local as a Global Remedy

L ARGE MULTINATIONAL CORPORATIONS profit from processed, mass-pro-duced and mass-marketed foods lacking in nutritional nourishment. Billions of boxes, cans and bags are filled with ingredients most of us cannot pronounce. Oftentimes, products from our modern food industry contain no real food ingredients. As a mother, what gets me the most is how big corporations are allowed to market artificially flavored and GMO foods packed with nothing but sugars and starches and virtually no nutritional value to kids! They know what kids like: sweet foods with bright colors and their favorite cartoon character on the box. This is a pretty genius marketing strategy but at whose expense? The poor children who are forced to sit still at school when their bodies are on a roller coaster of a sugar rush from their morning cereal. They get 15 minutes of fresh air on a concrete parking lot. No wonder so many children are diagnosed with ADHD and ADD. How could their tiny bodies sit still and concentrate after consuming over two grams of sugar, an assortment of food colorings and who knows how many hormones from the milk? Even as farmers who know what we should and shouldn't eat, my husband and I still succumb to the brilliant and deviant marketing strategies of the food giants. Seeing an "all natural" label next to a picture of a sunset over a farm or a barn usually brings comfort to all of us who have trust in companies that claim the word "natural." Much to my dismay, I learned that the term "all natural" is loosely regulated and that just because something is marketed as all natural doesn't mean that it is healthy. Additionally, along with the commercialization of organic foods comes a lapse in regulations, especially when organic regulations in other countries may be less strict than in the United States. This results in serious gray areas in terms of labeling for "natural" and "organic" foods. That's just the beginning. It's easy to forget that marketing strategies are implemented by the corporations themselves, not the FDA and not the EPA. For example, when I think of cage-free chickens, I think of happy-go-lucky chickens roaming on a beautiful farm. Cage-free actually means that they are just not in individual cages. They are still inside a huge warehouse, packed so tightly they can barely move.

Profit farms focus primarily on food production for profit, with virtually no reverence for soil health or water quality. They have led to soil degradation, erosion, pollution, groundwater contamination, deforestation and barren soil.

Factory farms, called CAFOs or concentrated animal feeding operations, raise cattle, chickens, pigs and other animals for food. Most often, they live in conditions that are unhealthy and unnatural so as to increase the company's profit margin. Crowded facilities have little access to fresh air and sunshine. Most are fed genetically modified (GM) grains, not their natural diet. Because they are given antibiotics, the meat contains disease-resistant bacteria. Ducks, lambs, geese, rabbits and turkeys may also be raised in these types of dense, highly populated factory farms. (Foodandwaterwatch.org)

Conventional farms use synthetic pesticides and fertilizers and often till the soil with heavy machinery on one hundred-plus acres of land.

Grain farms, such as commercial wheat farms, typically cover hundreds or even thousands of acres. Sadly, most wheat, the staple grain in flour production, is grown with the use of dangerous pesticides and fertilizers.

Unfortunately, the damage done by these farms has caused irreversible destruction to the environment. Fortunately, there are many large-scale farmers who are transitioning to no-till methods, more humane treatment of animals, pesticide-free growing methods and smaller-scale operations. Joel Salatin has been planting the way by offering practical advice for farmers who wish to make the transition from conventional farming to no-till farming.

I love the way biodynamic farmer Bobbi Sandwich puts it: "Farm animals need fresh air and sunshine to thrive. They need to scratch in the dirt and roll in the mud. They need space to roam." Bobbi and Alex, formerly of Live Springs Farm, are longtime real-food advocates and continuously educate their community about the importance of animal health and well-being. They have been farming using regenerative practices for over a decade. I truly admire their stewardship toward the land.

Luckily, thanks to real-food producers and consumers and inspirational figures in the Food Revolution such as Alice Waters, Barbara Kingsolver, Winona LaDuke, Vandana Shiva, Terry Bryant, Malik Yakini, Robyn O'Brien, Michael Pollan, Morgan Spurlock, Tyrone Hayes, Jamie Oliver, Robert Kenner, Joel Salatin, Will Allen, Robyn O'Brien and Cesar Chavez, individuals around the globe are becoming more and more informed about what is in their food and why it is important to read labels and buy locally.

Why Organic?

The term "organic" is defined as archaic or instrumental or forming an integral element of a whole. Organic gardening or farming means growing or producing without artificial chemical pesticides, herbicides, fungicides or fertilizers. To be truly organic is to go beyond the USDA's reductionist concept of organic. The USDA's guidelines for organic certification simply replaces synthetic applications with organic ones. These farms are of course making a good transition, but many still practice techniques that are harming the living components in the soil. Large-scale organic farms, while in my opinion a far better alternative to conventional farms, are still tilling the soil with large steel tines, causing irreversible damage in some parts of the world. They are still using an insane amount of water in areas where drought is prevalent. For example, large-scale certified organic farms in California are pumping in thousands of gallons of water.

In an ideal world, organic food would simply be called "food," and the non-organic food would be labeled with a big red sticker that says "contains enormous amounts of pesticides." In an ideal world, GMO foods would be labeled everywhere. In an ideal world, small family farms using regenerative farming techniques would feed their communities, limiting the need for large-scale industrialized farming. Beyond the organic label lies infinite possibilities for contributing to the organic movement (the original method of growing food). The possibilities all surround the self-sufficiency model and the idea of literally getting back to our roots. What if everyone knew how to grow their own food? What if every neighborhood had a community garden? What if every street corner had a produce stand?

A natural, organic philosophy will open your life in many healthy directions. The benefits of incorporating this philosophy into your garden as well as your life are endless. You may find yourself ...

⊛ observing the natural world and its harmony and balance

⊛ aligning yourself to the Earth's natural rhythms

⊛ letting go of synthetic sprays in your garage and household

⊛ consuming smarter and less

⊛ making healthy lifestyle choices

⊛ feeling better in your body

Organic is better for the environment! Humans have been growing organically up until the 20th century, when chemicals developed in the wake of the two world wars led to the "Green Revolution." The Green Revolution was not actually very green, and unfortunately these new growing methods, which quickly became the norm in industrialized nations, led to a devastating loss of healthy topsoil that had been built up over millennia. Pesticides, herbicides and fungicides (etc.) contaminate our groundwater with toxins that are harmful to our bodies, especially for children who are particularly vulnerable. The chemicals in many EPA-approved pesticides have been linked to cancer and other diseases. According to the Pesticide-Induced Diseases Database created by the Beyond Pesticides organization:

> The common diseases affecting the public's health are all too well-known in the 21st century: asthma, autism and learning disabilities, birth defects and reproductive dysfunction, diabetes, Parkinson's and Alzheimer's diseases, and several types of cancer. Their connection to pesticide exposure continues to strengthen despite efforts to restrict individual chemical exposure, or mitigate chemical risks, using risk assessment-based policy.

Many Americans are unaware of these harmful effects because the burdens of these toxic exposures are unequally borne by those who cannot choose to live or work far from these toxic industrial farms. Organic growing methods, on the other hand, promote healthy soils, ecosystems and human communities.

Plus, organic produce tastes better and contains many more nutrients than conventionally grown produce!

Beyond Organic

In 2010, my husband and I were hired on as the farmers at La Vista CSA Farm, my husband as the head farmer and myself as his field assistant/greenhouse supervisor. We jumped right into farming a diverse array of vegetables without pesticides on five acres on the bluffs of the Mississippi River. Where fertile soil meets changing seasons, we began a beautiful journey in the miraculous seed-to-table process of growing food for families.

From the moment I began planting thousands of seeds in the greenhouse that spring, it dawned on me that eating is one of the most profound human experiences; it not only is vital to our existence as our form of energy, but also defines us culturally. Food is tied to our culture, values and religious traditions. It doesn't just sustain us but holds our entire existence together. Waking hours are determined by our next meals, where we gather as a family or community to eat. Sharing a meal is one of the most universal forms of socialization, and many cultures revere the act as nearly sacred. In the Levant, special meals akin to Thanksgiving are regular family occurrences. In Spain, families and friends spend hours together at dinner. In certain parts of Spain, most businesses close between 1 pm and 4 pm to go home for *comida*, a midday meal at 2 pm and a very important family gathering time. In most parts of India, families share all meals together because it is thought that eating together strengthens the family bond.

In many cultures, food has a spiritual context. Their common thread is that food is offered to God first. For example, in Hare Krishna, a branch of Hinduism, food is offered to Krishna first to demonstrate devotion and gratitude. Similarly, offering food to Buddha is one of the oldest rituals documented in Buddhism and teaches the art of selfless love.

In addition to its cultural aspects, food can also affect us individually, altering our moods by positive or negative experiences as our taste buds carry information to our brains via the cranial nerves. This remarkable function can evoke memories based on taste alone. What we distinguish as taste is actually comprised 90 percent of smell. We are wired with the great ability to heartily enjoy what we eat. So why not enjoy food grown locally and responsibly, prepared lovingly and shared with those we love the most? Historically, food has been healthy and natural, not loaded and processed with pesticides, artificial flavors, preservatives, synthetic ingredients and food coloring. We may have more food than ever before, but if our food is not good for us, we are sacrificing a great deal of our health, money, longevity and pleasure.

While my husband and I are passionate about growing food for the families in our community, we know that farming is not sustainable. Small-scale farming is a better alternative to commercial farming, but it is still not the best practice for the soil. We do implement cover cropping, crop rotation, soil-building on perennials, companion planting and heavy mulching with nutrient-rich organic material, but we are still tilling the soil because that is the infrastructure that was in place before we arrived. Our individual goals are to teach others, especially children, how to grow their own food using permaculture techniques, soil-building, raised beds and water retention. We long to get back to our roots of no-till vegetable growing, and we are making steps to implement more and more of that during our time at La Vista.

Our long-term goal is to start an eco-retreat center and a permaculture teaching farm where individuals can come from around the world. Throughout the season, we offer workshops to community members and teach a gardening summer camp at our kids' school. We host several groups of children from The Nature Institute summer camp, teaching them about healthy soil and non-invasive growing techniques. They tour our permaculture orchard, compost pile and vermicompost system. They harvest their own green beans and cherry tomatoes, eat right from the plant and pull weeds with us. It becomes a day of hands-on learning that will stick with them for a long time. Groups of college students, who come for days of community service, make a huge difference in the workload and leave feeling accomplished and inspired by the good work they did to help a local farm family. By engaging with our community, we are setting a positive example of the tremendous impact eating locally can have on our health and the health of the environment. Food brings the community together.

According to Toby Hemenway's Permaculture Flower (modified from David Holmgren's), it is best to grow our own food in our own backyard first. What we can't grow ourselves, we can acquire at local community gardens and small farms or by supporting local farmers' markets. We can then support area businesses that sell local foods. Finally, only when we simply have used all our local resources, we visit the chain supermarket to complete our needs. This mindset offers a creative insight into how our thoughts about food need to shift a little in order to be truly invested in the local foods movement. Beyond food, the Permaculture Flower offers a solution-based concept that examines that big picture in all aspects of life, how basic human needs are interconnected and how to attain these needs while considering sustainability. We will dig into permaculture principles more in Chapter Three.

The world is painted with a beautiful oasis of rooftop gardens, backyard gardens, urban farms, community gardens, CSA farms and small family farms. With such abundance, there are plenty of avenues to meet the needs of aspiring and seasoned locavores. In any major city, one can find a plethora of local businesses that support local farmers. Supporting local food systems reduces our carbon footprint, circulates funds back into the local economy and promotes an understanding of the complexity of food: where it comes from, how it is grown, who was involved in production and delivery, where it is transported, how it was delivered, where it ends up, who cooks it, who gets to eat it and what it costs and why.

Though the local foods movement and conscious eating seems to be a modern-day trend, the concept is nothing new. The idea of "local foods" began over one million years ago with the first hunters and gatherers eating only what they could find in a 100-mile radius. It is only through the globalization of trade and the development of food industry technologies that the concept of local foods was lost to most of us. The modern local foods movement peaked during the victory garden days of World War I and II, when canning and preserving fruits and vegetables was the citizen's duty to reduce pressure on the public food supply during wartime. It took a long hiatus during the Industrial Revolution through the growth of grocery store chains in the 1950s.

Coincidently, the Green Revolution, which started during the 1950s and '60s, was the name given to the industrialization of mass food production prompted by the modernization of large-scale farming and the introduction of chemical fertilizers and pesticides, spawned from the development and production of war chemicals. While the Green Revolution may have begun as a way to help with starvation, it evolved into something far from it. Wouldn't it have been easier to pass laws requiring people nationwide to have space to grow their own food? For over five decades, junk food, convenience foods and prepackaged meals made their way onto kitchen tables around the world, and unfortunately that trend only grows as people get busier. Gardens were replaced with lawns. Real fruit was replaced with artificially flavored vacuum-packed fruit cups swimming in syrup. Home-cooked meals were replaced with Hamburger Helper. Commercials targeted women in the workforce, advertising promises of affordable and convenient meals for busy families.

Today, the local foods movement is back and here to stay! Gardening and self-sufficiency are hip again, and we are, in essence, getting back to our roots. While local foods may be slightly more expensive, it helps to think in terms of spending a bit more to reduce our overall healthcare costs and to improve our environment. Local foods grown without pesticides improve our health and are a viable form of preventative healthcare. Spending more to grow food using sustainable practices also contributes to the future of the planet. Localized food systems significantly lower the carbon footprint by reducing the distance that food travels and circulate funds back into the local economy. There are plenty of farmers' markets that accept SNAP benefits or food stamps, expanding access for low-income families. Locavores on a budget can join CSA farms and supplement with their own garden. The rise of food awareness is paramount for our growth as a healthy, sustainable community. Seeing the world from the potato's-eye view makes us firm believers in the local foods movement as a remedy to the global food crisis.

By teaching and empowering others, especially youth, to grow their own food, we provide them with a sense of purpose, personal accomplishment and responsibility. By encouraging them to source food locally, we instill in them a sense of community that fosters respect and commitment and provides a stepping-stone for them to tackle other concerns, such as deforestation, global climate change, air and water quality, natural gas fracking and exploitative extractive industries.

Know Your Farmer, Know Your Food

Luckily, we know plenty of farmers and are so grateful to be a part of a dynamite network of growers in the St. Louis Region. Some of our favorite farms in the Midwest are Bellews Creek Farm, Riverbend Roots, Three Rivers Community Farm, Live Springs Farm, Urban Buds, EarthDance Farms, Claverach Farm, Ozark Forest Mushrooms, Seeds of Hope Farm, New Roots Urban Farm, Food Roof STL and Such and Such Farm.

Ways you can support local farms in your community:

Grow a garden, join a community garden, shop at your local farmers' market or become a member at a CSA farm and see for yourself the value of eating locally grown produce! Farms are usually open to scheduled visits, open houses or public farm tours throughout the season.

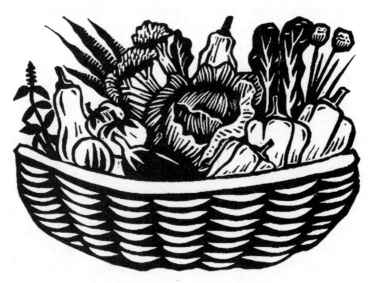

"Food Sustains Us; Let's Source Sustainable Foods": 8 Ways to Access Healthy Fresh Food

Without food, we could not exist.

1) Learn about permaculture as a global solution to food-related environmental, social and economic issues. Permaculture gardens utilize the existing landscape and produce food in harmony with each specific ecosystem. They focus on no-till methods with an emphasis on soil health, water preservation, companion planting and permaculture food forests. See Chapter Three.

2) Start your own container or square-foot garden to ease you into the art of growing food. Easy and affordable, container gardening requires very little space and is low maintenance, making it perfect for busy individuals. See Chapter Six.

3) Start your own backyard garden. It requires only a small amount of time and energy, especially using raised beds, which need little weeding. Wicking beds are cheap, low-maintenance garden beds composed of reclaimed materials. Backyard gardens attract pollinators and offer food for the entire family. See Chapter Four.

4) Start a food revolution by talking to your neighbors about starting frontyard gardens, which allow a highly sustainable food shed within your square block. Neighbors then share a diverse array of fresh vegetables. This idea builds community and creates safer, more vibrant neighborhoods. (See interview with John VanDeusen, founder of the Food Is Free Project. Page 236)

5) Start or join a community garden, an amazing opportunity for a diverse group of individuals to come together with the goal of growing healthy and fresh food. Most community garden plots are either free or require a small annual fee. According to the American Community Garden Association, "There are an estimated 18,000 community gardens throughout the United States and Canada alone." Community gardens worldwide offer excellent models for education and outreach, beautiful examples of how individuals from all walks of life in the same community can unite and bring a vision to fruition with love and support.

6) Volunteer on a farm. Find out which farms closest to you welcome volunteers or do work exchange. Contact the farmer directly about how you can help. WWOOF (Worldwide Opportunities on Organic Farms, wwoof.net) is an excellent resource for helping small farmers.

7) Join a CSA farm. Under a subscription model, shareholders or members pay upfront to help the small farmer with seed and operating costs and share in the risks and the benefits with the farmer. They receive a weekly share of the seasonal harvest grown throughout an allotted period of time, typically 26 weeks. Some CSA programs are available by the week instead of requiring an upfront seasonal cost. Others require or suggest that members volunteer on the farm in addition to paying a subscription fee.

8) Shop at your local farmers' market. Farmers' markets offer weekly (sometimes bi-weekly) opportunities to purchase fresh locally grown produce, dairy, eggs, meat and prepared foods at reasonable yet fair prices for the farmers. Fruits and vegetables are at their peak flavor and freshness, typically harvested just a few days earlier. Generally speaking, the farmers who grow the produce are the market vendors, which allows them to meet and shake hands with their customers.

9) Support local businesses that source from local farmers. Businesses dedicated to promoting and supporting small family farmers are popping up all over the world. Co-ops and family-owned health food stores typically stock produce only grown within a 150-mile radius. Local Harvest and local Slow Food USA chapters are resources for finding businesses in your area that support local foods.

There are many methods of indoor growing in a temperature-controlled environment using grow lights. Aeroponics, a very fast method, uses air and nutrient-rich water. Plants are misted regularly. Hydroponics is similar, but the plants are grown in a liquid nutrient-rich growing medium. Aquaponics uses water and the waste produced by fish, typically tilapia, which are also raised for food. These are all excellent ways to grow food in densely populated urban areas.

I prefer for the rain to fall softly upon the fields, upon the resilient plants whose roots are deep and whose stems stretch for the sun. There is something to be said about eating plants whose energy comes directly from the sun.

Types of Farms

Orchards grow fruit trees of one or several varieties, oftentimes remaining within families for generations. There are plenty of pick-your-own orchards throughout the United States. The main two orchard crops that grow in the Midwest are peaches in the summer and apples in the fall.

Specialized farms stick to one crop that thrives in that region. For example, there are many specialized lavender farms flourishing in distinctive climates worldwide. I highly recommend visiting a lavender farm; the views are stunning, the pollinators are plentiful and the scent is delightful.

Victory gardens were planted by citizens at home during World War I and II to promote self-sufficiency rather than reliance on food from the surrounding regions. It was also used as a way to lift the spirits of those affected by the war.

Biodynamic farms grow grains used to feed their animals, which are allowed to graze in the pasture. In return, the fields are fertilized with manure and compost. Soil health is a key component in biodynamic farming. Our friends Alex and Bobbi grow organic non-GMO grains and legumes. Their pigs, cows and chickens have plenty of room to roam, graze and forage throughout the open pastures and wooded areas.

Organic farms, which can be certified or non-certified, may use sustainable farming practices. However, not all certified organic farms are good for the environment. For example, many large-scale (150-plus acre) certified organic farms grow one single crop. Although these farms practice under the organic certification umbrella, they are still a monoculture, with one specific crop that uses up large quantities of minerals and elements from the soil. Large-scale commercial farms also use a lot of water, which can be harmful to the water table during a drought. Tilling the soil on these large farms kills the important beneficial bacteria and fungi in the soil. While these practices may not be the best for the environment, they are certainly better than conventional industrial methods. Every little small step is a step in the right direction. Organic is a better choice than non-organic, but growing your own food and sourcing from local farmers are still better choices than shopping at grocery stores, where produce is usually conventionally grown on large monoculture farms around the world. The best option would be if everyone had a no-till permaculture garden in their front- or backyard and shared the labor and harvest with neighbors. Luckily, we are seeing more and more such realities emerging.

According to Kris and Stacey Larson of Riverbend Roots Farm, for a small-scale non-certified organic diversified vegetable farm, "crop diversity is key in terms of soil health." The various root structures of plants grow into different levels of the soil, working together to prevent erosion and using and adding various nutrients to the soil. When farming for both crop productivity and soil building, Kris gives precedence to planting a diverse array of vegetables, fruits, flowers and herbs, not only to please members and market customers, but also for ecological reasons: to diversify the nutrient demand, to diversify food sources for pollinators and to attempt to prevent buildup of disease organisms, including certain species of harmful bacteria and fungi. Most organic farms do not spray pesticides, herbicides and fungicides unless the sprays are OMRI-certified or made from natural ingredients. Some small-scale organic farms make their own compost with leaves, grass clippings and vegetable scraps. They practice crop rotation, cover cropping and mulching with straw to feed the soil rather than deplete its nutrients. Fabric weed barriers and row covers suppress weeds and protect crops from insect damage.

Non-certified organic farms typically practice the same techniques, but operating under a limited budget, they cannot afford the USDA Organic label licensing and certification fees.

Heirloom farms grow only heirloom varieties of fruits, vegetables, grains, legumes, flowers and herbs. They use seeds that have been preserved rather than modified.

Pick-your-own farms exist countrywide, usually growing fruit, such as apples or berries. This is an excellent opportunity for children and their parents to spend some time feeling the Earth beneath their feet, the wind in their hair and the sun on their backs as they pick the bounty together and get in touch with nature. One great way to experience a pick-your-own farm is to make it into a picnic.

Growing Takes Many Forms

Grow. Grow organically. Grow naturally. Grow without the use of harmful pesticides toxic to humans, the watershed, the soil and the environment. Grow fruits. Grow vegetables. Grow herbs. Grow medicine. Grow an orchard. Grow *native plants*. Grow *trees*. Grow *flowers*.

When you grow, you nourish your body. You are an advocate for the Earth. You shape the world inch by inch. You reduce your carbon footprint. You limit your reliance on fossil fuels. You create a habitat for pollinators. You feed nutrients back to the Earth. You provide nutrient-rich food to your children, your family and your friends. You inspire neighbors. You "become the change you wish to see in the world." (Gandhi)

Grow. Grow mentally. Grow physically. Grow spiritually. When you spend the effort on growing your own food and medicine, you shape the path you walk to one that yields an enriching and fulfilling sense of wonder and peace. Witnessing a seedling sprout from the tiniest seed is a miraculous life process that often gets overlooked. Knowing life exists beneath our feet on a thriving cyclical momentum is profound. Plants are brilliant with complexity, interconnectedness and amazing processes such as photosynthesis. Plants heal. Plants nurture, protect and give us everything we need to walk this Earth. Our connections to plants have been seriously hindered in the last few centuries. Throughout history, there have been cultures, tribes and individuals who valued and respected plants, who lived in harmony with their natural environments.

Grow. Grow friendships. Grow passion. Grow community. Grow neighborhoods. Grow community gardens. Grow urban farms. Grow rural farms. Grow family farms. Grow rooftop gardens. Grow on your balcony. Grow in your kitchen window. Grow food, not lawns.

If you already grow your own food using organic or sustainable methods, you understand the relationship to the soil, to your food. You are truly a steward of the Earth. Be sure to continuously acknowledge the fact that you are doing a remarkable job on this Earth. Feel free to skip the next few chapters, scan as a refresher course or pass them along to someone who has not yet discovered the fulfillment of growing.

Now that we have covered various types of farms and how you can become involved in food issues within your communities, you have choices to make about what is right for you and your family. Eating locally shifts your view on food and what to prepare when. Find out what grows locally during each month and ask farmers and neighbors how they prepare their produce. Check your local garden clubs for seed swaps, plant sharing and recipe ideas.

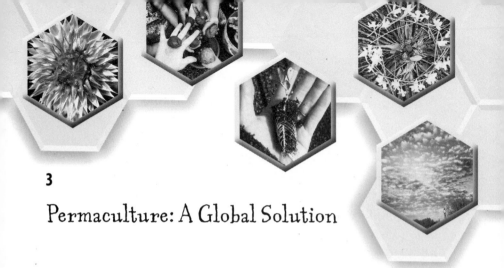

3

Permaculture: A Global Solution

PERMACULTURE CONCEPTS are at the heart of any sustainable endeavor. Understanding their vast potential to guide us toward a sustainable future is vital to creating a paradigm shift. We have a last chance at clean air, clean water and healthy soil, factors absolutely necessary for healthy survival. Permaculture can help us find ways that we, as individuals, can help heal the Earth and revitalize our air, water and soil.

In 1978, Bill Mollison and David Holmgren coined the term "permaculture" to stand for "permanent agriculture," but the word has since developed a second meaning: "permanent culture." Bill Mollison was an instructor, and David Holmgren was one of his undergraduate students. The book *Permaculture One* started out as David's undergraduate thesis. Bill developed a more hands-on approach to permaculture while David focused on theories and broad perspective potential in permaculture. Both are equally revered as leading permaculture experts, but Bill is deemed the "Father of Permaculture." He founded the Permaculture Institute in Tasmania to teach permaculture principles through hands-on education. In *Introduction to Permaculture*, he outlines the major principles: relative location, multiple functions, multiple elements, energy-efficient planning, using biological resources, energy cycling, small-scale intensive, accelerating succession, diversity, edge awareness and attitudinal principles. Bill Mollison planted the way for hundreds of permaculturists. He laid the foundation for Earth stewardship and is a hero among so many who wish to leave the world better than they found it.

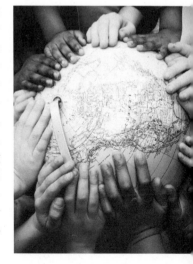

Permaculture begins with looking at the world through hopeful eyes, picturing a reality in which people attempt to work in harmony with the Earth, rather than against it. To look to nature for inspiration is a great way to truly absorb and observe the importance of biodiversity. For example, a native pollinator garden next to a vegetable garden promotes a symbiotic relationship between plants and pollinators. Our plates would be empty without pollinators. Channeling and preserving water significantly reduces water waste, helps to retain moisture so your garden thrives. Building your home with natural materials found on your building site reduces your reliance on synthetic and nonrenewable building materials, and is more energy efficient and very cost-effective. Building berms and swales allows for the channeling and preservation of water around a specific grouping of trees or crops. A berm is essentially a raised bed made from organic materials, and a swale is a specialized ditch that acts as a water preservation reservoir. Rainwater collected in the swale is redirected into the channels where it slowly and passively enters the soil.

Punta Mona Center for Sustainable Living and Education

In 1999, I went on a high-school trip to the rainforest of Costa Rica. We visited the Punta Mona Center for Sustainable Living and Education, an 85-acre organic permaculture farm on the Caribbean coast, run by eco-entrepreneur Stephen Brooks. He and his sister Lisa started Costa Rican Adventures to educate international students about rainforest degradation, endangered species and unsustainable agricultural practices, as well as solutions to these concerns. We visited the banana plantations where planes sprayed pesticides on the trees, causing nearby villages to suffer through the clouds of chemicals. We then visited the BriBri tribe at Kekoldi Indigenous Reserve in Puerto Viejo de Talamanca. They had been growing cacao trees for several generations in the understory of their food forests. They hand-ground the cacao and mixed it with tapa dulce, blocks of raw sugar. Walking through their food forest, witnessing such a diversity of tropical fruit trees among the jungle backdrop is memory etched in the catacombs of my mind. The BriBri tribe had a deep unparalleled connection with their food.

We witnessed the entire process of making chocolate: the pods were harvested from the trees; the pods were sliced open and the pulp removed; the beans were sorted, fermented and dried in the sun. A respected grandmother in the tribe, whose hands were worn from years of hard physical labor, kissed each and every dried cacao bean before she ground the seeds by hand using a stone corn grinder. A rich drink was made using fresh goat's milk, hot water, raw sugar and ground cacao. Each sip was magic. The process was beautiful. I was able to shake the hands of each member of the smiling BriBri tribe who worked so hard to make this one cup of hot chocolate. They sold the chocolate in a four-inch roll, with six disks of rich chocolate wrapped in wax paper. The aroma was earthy and robust. The taste was authentic, bold, bitter and sweet all at once. This experience forever shaped my love and appreciation not only for chocolate but also for all the hands of all the farmers whose hearts were committed to growing good food without pesticides. It certainly broadened my awareness of the importance of buying fair-trade and direct-trade chocolate. The experience of exploring through the cloud forests and jungles and along coastlines of Costa Rica reaffirmed my love for the natural world and helped to strengthen the desire to do my part for the Earth.

Stephen, also the founder of Kopali Organics, an organic food company dedicated to supporting small farmers and providing a highly nutritious food source to the public, has been a major catalyst in the permaculture movement. He has taught thousands of individuals around the globe how to bring sustainability into fruition in their daily lives. Punta Mona is completely off the grid, using solar energy for power, methane for gas and growing 90 percent of the food for thousands of people per year at the retreat center. The property is rich with biodiversity; hundreds of fruit and nut trees tower over a food forest and dozens of raised beds in the kitchen garden. Several types of squash thrive on the hillsides. Chinampas, wetland gardens, are home to various fruits, vegetables, roots, leaves and herbs. It is one of the most beautiful permaculture design models I have seen.

During my stay at Punta Mona, I learned the following ten central concepts of permaculture:

1. Permaculture incorporates the existing ecosystem into the development plans without compromising the integrity of the land, water or habitat of native flora and fauna.

2. Permaculture works with nature, not against it.

3. Permaculture gardens provide food for humans, animals, pollinators and the soil.

4. Permaculture fosters symbiotic relationships.

5. Permaculture provides a global solution to widespread epidemics, including hunger and starvation, environmental degradation, deforestation, pollution and reliance on fossil fuels.

6. Permaculture gardens help heal the land and its people by using plants to filter water, revitalizing contaminated soil, using grey water systems, implementing rain garden techniques, cultivating with the contours of the land and growing more per square foot.

7. Permaculture promotes all aspects of sustainability and focuses on how all solutions for a greener future can work together. Integrating alternative energy systems into small-scale organic food production is just one way to implement these concepts.

8. Permaculture promotes healthy food, clean air and clean water.

9. Permaculture focuses on the complex interrelationships within the food web and restores our balance with the natural world.

10. Permaculture is a catalyst for a sustainable future. Everyone is capable of practicing permaculture techniques.

Toby Hemenway offers a beautiful definition of permaculture:

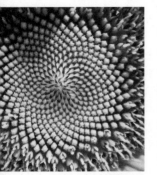

"I think the definition of permaculture that must rise to the top is that it is a design approach to arrive at solutions, just as the scientific method is an experimental approach. In more concrete terms, permaculture tells how to choose from a dauntingly large toolkit — all the human technologies and strategies for living — to solve the new problem of sustainability. It is an instruction manual for solving the challenges laid out by the new paradigm of meeting human needs while enhancing ecosystem health. The relationship explicitly spelled out in that view, which connects humans to the larger, dynamic environment, forces us to think in relational terms, which is a key element of permaculture. The two sides of the relationship are explicitly named in two permaculture ethics: care for the Earth, and care for people. And knowing we need both sides of that relationship is immensely helpful in identifying the problems we need to solve.

First, what are human needs? The version of the permaculture flower that I work with names some important ones: food, shelter, water, waste recycling, energy, community, health, spiritual fulfillment, justice and livelihood. The task set out by permaculture, in the new paradigm, is to meet those needs while preserving ecosystem health, and we have metrics for assessing the latter. The way those needs are met will vary by place and culture, but the metrics of ecosystem health can be applied fairly universally. This clarifies the task set by permaculture, and I think it also distinguishes permaculture from the philosophy — the paradigm — required to use it effectively and helps us understand why permaculture is often called a movement. Permaculturists make common cause with all the other millions of people who are shifting to the new paradigm, and it is that shift — not the design approach of permaculture that supports it — that is worthy of being called a movement. Permaculture is one approach used by this movement to solve the problems identified by the new paradigm. To do this, it operates on the level of strategies rather than techniques, but that is a subject for another essay. Because we are, in a way, still in the phlogiston era of our ecological awareness, we don't know how to categorize permaculture, and we can confuse it with the paradigm that it helps us explore. Permaculture is not the movement of sustainability and it is not the philosophy behind it; it is the problem-solving approach the movement and the philosophy can use to meet their goals and design a world in which human needs are met while enhancing the health of this miraculous planet that supports us."

— Toby Hemenway.

This image illustrates a comprehensive solution-based example of how a paradigm shift can create a world that works for everyone. It focuses on equality, environmental intelligence, spiritual awakening, food and resource localization, community building and a unified desire for positive change. What if this could be implemented worldwide? Think of the possibilities!

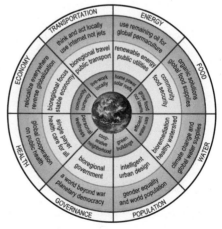

From a Bay Area Permaculture Group brochure, published in *West Coast Permaculture News & Gossip and Sustainable Living Newsletter* (Fall 1995).

Permaculture Ethics, Principles, Attitudes and Rules

The following is reproduced with permission from Toby Hemenway:

Permaculture Ethics

1. Care for the Earth
2. Care for people
3. Return the surplus

Primary Principles for Functional Design

1. Observe. Use protracted and thoughtful observation rather than pro-longed and thoughtless action. Observe the site and its elements in all seasons. Design for specific sites, clients and cultures.
2. Connect. Use relative location: Place elements in ways that create useful relationships and time-saving connections among all parts. The number of connections among elements creates a healthy, diverse ecosystem, not the number of elements.
3. Catch and store energy and materials. Identify, collect and hold useful flows. Every cycle is an opportunity for yield, every gradient (in slope, charge, heat, etc.) can produce energy. Reinvesting resources builds capacity to capture yet more resources.
4. Each element performs multiple functions. Choose and place each element in a system to perform as many functions as possible. Beneficial connections between diverse components create a stable whole. Stack elements in both space and time.
5. Each function is supported by multiple elements. Use multiple methods to achieve important functions and to create synergies. Redundancy protects when one or more elements fail.
6. Make the least change for the greatest effect. Find the "leverage points" in the system and intervene there, where the least work accomplishes the most change.
7. Use small-scale, intensive systems. Start at your doorstep with the smallest systems that will do the job, and build on your successes, with variations. Grow by chunking.

Principles for Living and Energy Systems

8. Optimize edge. The edge — the intersection of two environments — is the most diverse place in a system and is where energy and materials accumulate or are transformed. Increase or decrease edge as appropriate.

9. Collaborate with succession. Systems will evolve over time, often toward greater diversity and productivity. Work with this tendency, and use design to jump-start succession when needed.

10. Use biological and renewable resources. Renewable resources (usually living beings and their products) reproduce and build up over time, store energy, assist yield and interact with other elements.

Attitudes

11. Turn problems into solutions. Constraints can inspire creative design. "We are confronted by insurmountable opportunities." — Pogo (Walt Kelly)

12. Get a yield. Design for both immediate and long-term returns from your efforts: "You can't work on an empty stomach." Set up positive feedback loops to build the system and repay your investment.

13. The biggest limit to abundance is creativity. The designer's imagination and skill limit productivity and diversity more than any physical limit.

14. Mistakes are tools for learning. Evaluate your trials. Making mistakes is a sign you're trying to do things better.

Rules for Resource Use

Ranked from regenerative to degenerative, different resources can:

1. increase with use
2. be lost when not used
3. be unaffected by use
4. be lost by use
5. pollute or degrade systems with use

These principles are designed to be implemented into permaculture design projects and can apply to growing gardens, food forests and farms in eco-villages. These plans and ideas can be scaled down or scaled up and are good guidelines to follow in any planting or community-building endeavor. Permaculture techniques work especially well in areas with low annual rainfall. When implemented correctly, these techniques are meant to be resilient and long-lasting. Some take more time to create but later require less labor for a high yield.

Growers around the globe help heal themselves, their communities and their environment by bringing permaculture to life one seed at a time. The essence of permaculture is the ability to understand the symbiotic relationships between people and people, plants and people, plants and the Earth, and food production and the environment. Paying homage to each other as stewards of the Earth by offering support and encouragement is one way we can truly send out ripples of change to the world.

Real food grown from the Earth is the very point where all these relationships intersect. Throughout cultural history everywhere, the connection human beings have had to the land and to their food has deepened by being in tune with nature and the changing seasons. For example, certain civilizations held grains, vegetables, fruits, nuts and seeds as sacred. Rituals, ceremonies and celebrations were held during planting and harvesting.

Bridging the gap between cultural diversity and biodiversity is a key component in permaculture. Understanding the complexity of nature's resilience and strength gives us a model to learn from. Sharing these observations with growers worldwide is very important for the future of the planet. We can inspire and teach each other based on our own observations. From witnessing a dandelion plant grow through the cracks of concrete to seeing a redwood tree sapling emerge from a clear-cut, we have so much to learn from nature. Cultivation methods have been passed down through scriptures, scrolls and oral traditions. Innovative ways of growing food seem to be more prevalent today than ever because of social media. More people are experimenting with home gardening. Once you delve into the art of growing food, you discover so many other possible endeavors, including herb-growing for medicine, food preservation, wild-edible foraging, wild crafting, beer making, beekeeping and animal husbandry. Growing food then becomes this momentous act with the potential to define the rest of one's life course. It was for me anyway. It brings about feelings of liberation and independence that are unmatched, empowering me to rely less and less on industrialized food systems.

Practice Permaculture in Your Own Backyard

Grow an organic vegetable garden to feed your family, friends and neighbors. Use straw to mulch or practice lasagna gardening and sheet mulching to suppress weeds. Integrate a food forest into your existing landscape.

Plant perennial fruits and fruit trees.

Get a rain barrel and use a rainwater catchment system to water your garden. Build simple bioswales to channel water.

Start a compost pile to produce your own organic fertilizer and reduce waste. Build your soil by adding organic matter.

Plant native perennial flowers to attract pollinators. Plant native trees to clean the air and provide a wildlife habitat.

Permaculture can be easily implemented in relationships and in spiritual practice in terms of healing the self and living in symbiosis with each other. Acknowledging strengths in others is a vital aspect; encouraging, uplifting and inspiring each other to work toward common goals and for the greater good is a necessity in the paradigm shift. Unconditional love and reverence for all earths ecology replaces the ego and competitive nature. After all, anyone involved in permaculture is ultimately striving for the same goal and is working toward the greater good. Practicing gratitude is also an instrument for positive change.

A Permaculture Poem

In dwellings around the globe, individuals are awakening to a calling greater than themselves.

From urban city apartments to humble abodes at the foothills of magnificent mountains ... people are waking up

From flats in Ireland to huts in Ghana ... people are waking up

From highrises near the equator to low valleys in the southern hemisphere ... people are waking up

From the banks of the Mighty Mississippi to the shores of the Caribbean Sea ... people are waking up

We feel an innate connection to the Earth in our hearts. We see the damage that has been done, and we realize the need for change. As a collective response to Earth's wound that we have witnessed, many of us are uniting to create a paradigm shift. Our collective consciousness is expanding. We are always evolving and developing. But without permaculture, we stop healing, we stop caring, and the wound deepens.

As individuals with the beautiful gifts of free will, creativity and passion, we have a major advantage. We have infinite resources available at our fingertips — within ourselves and in our communities. The collective knowledge of past and present communities is abundant and free-flowing, if one simply knows where to look for it.

With these gifts, we can make a difference. We are making a difference.

Natural ecosystems have painted our Earth with beauty in the form of forests, deserts, prairies, wetlands, mountains, valleys, rivers, oceans, glaciers. The "green hearts" of our time are creating new works of art on our Earth: prairie and wetland restorations, backyard gardens, fruit and nut orchards, community gardens, organic and biodynamic farms and permaculture villages, all of which are purifying our air, improving water quality, returning nutrients to the soil, providing food to families and creating habitats for pollinators.

In gardens worldwide, we are planting seeds of change in fields of hope. People from all walks of life are waking up to the importance of sustainability by reading, listening, reflecting, brainstorming solutions and enacting them.

We are getting back to our roots and respecting the land as ancient cultures did long ago. Being self-sufficient is no new endeavor, of course, but wading through the muck that the Industrial Revolution and mass consumption have left behind makes it seem new.

Permaculture Grounds Us with Possibilities for Positive Change

My husband and I have always dreamed of getting our permaculture certifications, but our finances and inability to spend a month away from our children have prevented us from doing so. However, this does not imply that we are incapable of bringing visions of permaculture into fruition in our own lives. In fact, it proves that anyone and everyone can practice permaculture techniques, with or without an official certification.

Welcoming Permaculture into Your Life

Pick A Manageable Permaculture Project to Implement

Perhaps your goal is to grow 70 percent of your own produce this year. Or maybe you would like to have a medicinal herb garden. Or, more generally, say you want to become more self-sufficient. Figuring out how a specific project designed with permaculture concepts can assist you with your personal goals is a wonderful place to start.

For example, this year, our goal is to integrate permaculture into the CSA farm we manage, starting with the orchard. With the help from local permaculture enthusiasts, we will install a bioswale along the perimeter to preserve and channel water, plant native flowers and shrubs to attract pollinators, mulch each tree with heavy compost to feed the soil and integrate alliums to deter pests. Bringing the basic concepts of permaculture into practice builds a strong foundation for growing as an ever-evolving art form.

Permaculture Books

There are several very well-written books, each tailored to specific learning styles, that are available at your library or from the authors. Permaculture creates paths of inspiration. Readers will follow the path that is right for them. Good books to start with include:

> Introduction to Permaculture by Bill Mollison
> Permaculture: Principles and Pathways Beyond Sustainability
>   by David Holmgren
> Gaia's Garden: A Guide to Home-Scale Permaculture
>   by Toby Hemenway
> The Permaculture Handbook by Peter Bane
> Restoration Agriculture by Mark Shepard
> Permaculture magazine

Start Your Personal Revolution in the Kitchen

Make a pledge to eat only fair-trade, organic, non-GM foods. Support your local small-scale farmers and businesses that try to be more sustainable in your community. Eliminating processed foods becomes a form of direct action. Inspiring friends and family to eat healthy foods becomes a step toward positive change. Growing your own fruits and vegetables and eating with the seasons become ways to reduce your carbon footprint.

Permaculture Networks

Start a permaculture network in your community or check social media for local groups or meet-ups to join. Get together often. Organize and host workshops. Work on projects together. Start a backyard revolution in your community.

Workplace Permaculture

Organize lunch potlucks or permaculture plantings at your workplace. Start a recycling program. Talk your organization into buying only green office supplies. Ask them to convert to greenware in the cafeteria.

Big City Permaculture

Get the youth involved by suggesting that teachers include permaculture projects and concepts in their curricula. They love new ideas for engaging students in the natural surroundings of their schools. Outdoor classrooms are more common than ever, and community service provides an excellent opportunity to get kids excited about growing food. Planting trees, installing vegetable gardens, building a rain garden and landscaping with native plants are just a few ways to implement simple permaculture concepts into the school grounds. Visit urban farms and community gardens. Volunteer in neighborhood plantings.

Permaculture Education

Learn online through websites or free courses. Research what options suit you best. The world is home to millions of permaculture enthusiasts. Use the internet to connect with others who are working on projects like yours.

Permaculture Conferences

Attending a conference is an excellent opportunity to meet like-minded individuals from around the world who are interested in permaculture.

Sustainability Starts from Within: Permaculture Brings the Vision into Fruition

Permaculture is a global solution to many environmental crises. In a household built around permaculture principles, you will find many useful supplies and resources:

- Mason jars in a variety of shapes and sizes
- Saved seeds that are accurately preserved and labeled
- Books on sustainability, including but not limited to permaculture, gardening, natural health, medicinal herbs, native plants and trees, wild edibles; books on tree, plant, bird and mushroom identification; textbooks from every class ever taken on ecology, biology, chemistry, geology and Earth science, etc.
- Magazines including *National Geographic*, *Mother Earth News*, *Permaculture* and *GRIT*, as well as every local publication that contains an article about gardening
- Reclaimed materials stockpiled for future building projects
- Dozens of jars of grains, nuts, seeds
- Homegrown canned fruits and veggies, jams and jellies, and staples including organic dried beans and grains
- Dried herbs for cooking, tea and medicine
- House plants for air purification and to keep you company when you must work inside
- Recycled everything, especially paper

- ⊕ A food dehydrator, a blender and a food processor, possibly pedal- or solar-powered
- ⊕ A teapot and a French press
- ⊕ A clothesline
- ⊕ An ongoing to-do list that is added to most likely every 15 minutes
- ⊕ A wood-burning stove and a stockpile of fallen wood
- ⊕ A dozen different journals
- ⊕ Handmade articles — furniture, clothing and pretty much handmade everything else
- ⊕ Various art and hobby supplies
- ⊕ A secret stash of fair-trade organic chocolate
- ⊕ An unbreakable spirit

Another one of my heroes is Winona LaDuke, a member of the Mississippi Band of Anishinaabe in Minnesota, an activist, author, mother and educator who works on issues of food sovereignty, indigenous environmental justice, and land recovery. She has been advocating for social and environmental change for decades and has made significant process in her community. She is the executive director of two nonprofits: Honor the Earth and the White Earth Land Recovery Project. Her work is a beautiful example of how vision can come to fruition with the support of the community and the ambition to see real change occur. Her spirit is unbreakable. Visit her website at www. nativeharvest.com

One of the most powerful quotes I have heard is, "Someone needs to explain to me why wanting clean drinking water makes you an activist and why proposing to destroy water with chemical warfare doesn't make you a terrorist." — Winona LaDuke

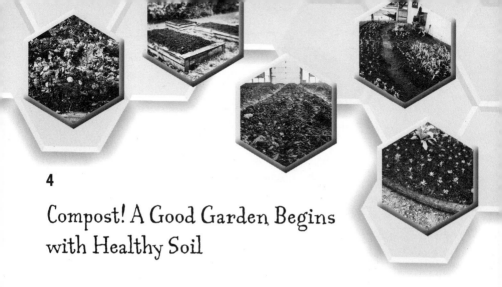

4

Compost! A Good Garden Begins with Healthy Soil

Healthy Soil, Healthy Plants

Q UALITY SOIL is the most vital aspect of growing organically! A healthy living soil is the key to vigorous and healthy plants. Compost, vermicompost and other organic soil supplements can add nutrients to your soil, improving plant vitality. As my husband, Eric, says, "Building healthy soil is the key to having optimal health in any garden setting. In can be thought of in terms of building the soil's immune system to help fight off unwanted diseases or pests."

All soils are different. A soil analysis or test is a good starting point to determine what nutrients might be lacking and to understand better its composition and personality. Midwest Bio-Ag provides soil analyses and creates custom natural fertilizers that are OMRI-certified based on their tests.

As sustainable farmers, we love our compost. We have seen the enormous difference that it makes on tomatoes, eggplant and peppers. We experimented by planting two rows of identical crops, one row with compost and one row without. The row with compost doubled in size within just a few short weeks.

Eric observed:

> In my 18 years of natural gardening and farming, there has always been a compost pile in the back corner somewhere. From the beginning of my adventures in gardening, I remember the exciting realization that over half of my waste can simply be thrown into a bin in a corner of my yard and over time would break down into the most nutrient-rich soil. To me, this concept became more and more fascinating as I noticed the similarities between what was happening in my compost bin and what was happening in nature. I would throw all of my veggie ends and recycled brown paper bags in the compost bin and forget about

it for months. When I turned the compost bin, I discovered the black gold that I had been reading about.

Ideally, all of our garden beds would be exactly like a compost bin, alive with various layers gently breaking down with no compaction.

We are often asked questions like, "How do you build healthy soil?" and "What can I add to my soil to make it organic?" Our answer is based on the same concept every time: the soil is a living, breathing organism covering the Earth's surface. Like all living things, it needs to be fed proper nutrients to thrive.

Nature is an excellent model to follow. We like to encourage individuals to look at nature, to really look. Observe the forest floor up close. Notice the layers of leaves, twigs, moss, fungi and detritus all decaying at various rates. You will notice the top layer has the appearance of basic mulch. Scratch the surface and you will notice the layers below get broken down inch by inch into perfect soil. We strive to obtain those rich qualities in the soil by mimicking those natural layers in the substances we add to our own garden soil.

Good garden soil is essentially a larger version of a compost pile. For example, a compost pile consists of materials that are in varying stages of decomposition. It also contains many organic materials from veggie scraps to leaf litter to grass clippings. Good garden soil, like a compost pile, contains an array of organic detritus with good aeration and good drainage.

Ideal garden soil is composed of ongoing layers of the following:

- Small stems and twigs
- Fallen leaves
- Grass clippings
- Compost
- Worm castings
- Aged sawdust (untreated)
- Living organisms
- Fruit and vegetable scraps
- Other organic matter

Vermiculture

Vermiculture is a fancy way to say worm farming, the use of worms to break down organic material. Its by-product is a nutrient-rich natural fertilizer called worm castings. Vermicompost is similar to compost, but it uses certain species of worms such as red wrigglers and earthworms to help break down organic material instead of simple heat, pressure and time. Purchase worms online, through mail order or at a bait shop. Bins can be kept in homes or classrooms.

Rich in nitrogen, phosphorus and potassium, vermicompost contains both macronutrients and micronutrients to benefit plant health and stimulate plant growth. It can also be made into a nutrient-rich "compost tea" that can be used to water garden plants. We use one part vermicompost to ten parts water. Simply fill a burlap sack, a potato sack or any mesh bag with vermicompost. Add the sack to a large bin, Rubbermaid container or 55-gallon drum and fill with water. Cover with fine mesh to prevent mesquitos. Steep the bag for one to seven days.

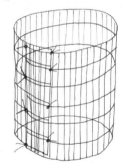

Worm castings, the final by-product of vermicompost, are the aggregate, dark brown, rich soil medium at the bottom of the bin. They can be added to a seed-starting soil mixture. Use worm castings to top-dress seedlings in pots, side-dress larger transplants and cover the tops of smaller beds.

Simple Compost Bin Designs Made from Reclaimed Materials

Although some compost bins cost hundreds of dollars, you don't need to spend that much on a new compost tumbler. Instead, use materials already available to you, waiting for a second life.

Wire Fence Cylinder Compost Bin

Use scrap wire fencing with holes no smaller than 2×4 inches. Use a panel about 10 feet long. Form a cylinder and fasten the ends together with bailing wire, overlapping the ends a few inches for extra support.

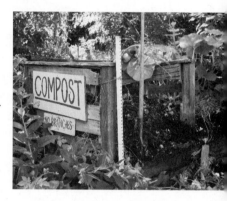
WIRE FENCE CYLINDER COMPOST BIN

Basic Cube Compost Bin

A simple compost bin can be made using reclaimed pallets, ones marked HT, meaning they have been treated with heat rather than chemicals. Securely fasten four pallets together upright with baling wire.

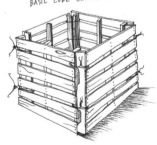
BASIC CUBE COMPOST BIN

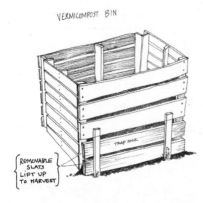

VERMICOMPOST BIN

TRAP DOOR

{ REMOVABLE SLATS LIFT UP TO HARVEST }

Vermicompost Bin

A vermicompost bin is like a compost bin except with worms added to break down materials more quickly. Worm castings can be harvested and used as organic fertilizer after about four months. Construct a vermicompost bin the same way with pallets, adding a trapdoor or removable slats to harvest worm castings.

For each design, put the fastened bin where you will keep it permanently in your yard, with an open end directly on the soil or grass. To best activate the composting process, fill the empty bin with leaves, grass clippings, straw and other organic matter. Then begin adding kitchen scraps such as vegetable and fruit ends and peels, egg shells and coffee grounds. Avoid adding meat, dairy, oils and citrus fruits. There is no need to turn compost in a vermiculture bin. The worms will do the work. Do not cover the compost bin. During dry spells, you may need to add water to your compost bin.

Permaculturist Aaron Jerad describes bacteria as "the smallest but most abundant member of the soil food web. Often feared but essential, whether directly or indirectly, for the survival of almost all other living organisms on Earth."

While backyard composting is not an exact science, it certainly adds beneficial bacteria and nutrients to your garden beds. However, when making your own compost at a larger scale, there are certain factors to keep in mind, such as maintaining temperature, regular turning for good air circulation and water drainage, and keeping weed seeds and plant pathogens at bay.

If you plan to compost at home, be sure you have a system in place. We use a small trash can with a pedal that lifts the lid. A five-gallon bucket with a lid works well, too. We empty ours every three days, and there is virtually no smell. If you would like a smaller option, any container with a lid would work, such as a one-gallon ice cream container. If you are worried about the smell, add a scoop of sawdust after each addition to the bin.

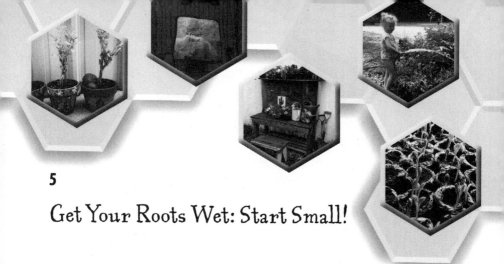

5

Get Your Roots Wet: Start Small!

W ITH JUST A FEW SIMPLE SUPPLIES and very little money, you can start growing your own food! A great place to start is your kitchen window.

Regrow Your Vegetable Scraps

Start in your kitchen window with your vegetable scraps, the cut ends of vegetables. Scallion and chive ends will regrow in soil continuously, as long as a small root section remains intact. Have fresh scallions and chives in your kitchen window year-round. Use a medium clay flowerpot with a small hole at the bottom. For good drainage and to prevent root rot, add a layer of small rocks or sand, then a nice mix of potting soil and compost. Place scallion ends root side down into the soil, pressing firmly so they are secure. Water once per week and watch them grow. Many vegetables will keep growing after they've been cut and planted in the same fashion and should be provided with appropriate amounts of water and sunlight.

- Bok choi
- Cabbage
- Celery
- Fennel
- Ginger
- Leeks
- Lettuce
- Onions
- Pineapple
- Scallions
- Sprouting garlic
- Sprouting potatoes
- Sprouting sweet potatoes

Some veggie scraps will regrow by simply placing the root end in water. Potatoes, sweet potatoes and ginger must be buried in soil.

Sprouting

Sprouts, which can be maintained year-round, are an excellent way to pack in those nutrients during the winter when fresh produce is unavailable, unless

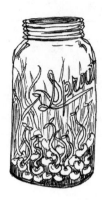

you have a backyard high-tunnel operation. Rich in phytonutrients, vitamins and minerals, sprouts are also an excellent source of protein for children. So, while you are waiting to transplant your vegetable starts, try growing some sprouts to snack on. Each has a unique flavor and nutritional profile. Sprouts, which are actually a living food, are said to be ten times more nutritious than some of the healthiest vegetables available.

Fenugreek sprouts have superb nutritional healing qualities and have been used to treat Type 2 diabetes. They are tangy and slightly bitter with a root-like taste, whereas lentil sprouts have more of a nutty, sweet earthy flavor. Lentil sprouts are an excellent source of protein and rich in calcium, iron and vitamins A and C. Mung bean sprouts are the typical bean sprouts found garnishing most Asian-inspired dishes and have a neutral fresh bean flavor. They are extremely high in vitamin K. Adzuki bean sprouts are also neutral with a slightly sharp aftertaste. Adzuki beans are a highly nutritious superfood. Broccoli, cabbage, radish and turnip sprouts are also extremely nutritious but typically require growing in a soil medium at home. Sunflower sprouts are in my opinion the most delicious sprouts; however, they typically require a growing medium and oftentimes don't produce as well or as quickly in a kitchen window as other kinds of sprouts. They are definitely worth the effort, though!

There are many ways to sprout! I prefer soaking seeds overnight in a Mason jar covered with cheesecloth. I rinse and drain the seeds each day and keep them in a sunny window. Within a few days, they have sprouted and are ready to eat. I like to sprout a few different varieties at once for a nice diversity of flavor, color, texture and nutrient density.

Purchase seeds online through Johnny's Selected Seeds, at most health food stores and some at grocery stores.

Basic Sprouting Directions

> Mason jars (one jar per variety)
> ½ cup of beans or 3 tablespoons seeds
> Enough water to fill a mason jar ¾ of the way full
> 5 × 5-inch square of fine cheesecloth per jar

In a wide-mouth quart-size Mason jar, add ½ cup of beans or 3 tablespoons seeds. Fill jar about ¾ full with purified water. Cover with a square of fine cheesecloth fastened with a rubber band. Soak overnight. In the morning, turn the jar upside down to drain the water through the cheesecloth. Rinse and drain twice after initial soaking. Store jar in a sunny window. Rinse and drain the seeds once or twice each day until they sprout, typically within a few days. Once sprouted, they are ready to eat. Always rinse sprouts well before eating. The bean and seed sprouts will continue to grow for a few days. They will stay fresh for a few days on the counter, but I like to rinse and dry them on day three of sprouting and store them in the refrigerator. It is best to consume sprouts within four or five days.

Sprouting is also a fun and easy edible science experiment for kids of all ages. Children get excited about food they take part in. Our whole family enjoys snacking on raw sprouts. They can be tossed in various spices such as smoked paprika and garlic and eaten as a snack. They also make delicious garnishes to soups and salads. A variety of sprouts can be combined to make a sprouted bean- and seed- salad. Add slices of your favorite veggies, a little vinaigrette, salt, cracked pepper and voila! You've got a delicious, fresh, homegrown winter salad.

Additionally, delicious nut milks can be made using soaked nuts and a high-powered blender. I recently made sprouted almond milk sweetened with the maple syrup that my husband made from sap collected from trees near the farm. I served the maple almond milk with raw chocolate truffle cookies, also made from sprouted almonds. That is one healthy snack that gets devoured immediately in our home.

Herbs

Herbs have been grown for centuries for both their culinary and medicinal properties. They are easy to cultivate and maintain in your kitchen window, on your balcony or in your yard. If you choose to grow herbs in your yard, I suggest three separate beds: one for perennials, one for annuals and one for medicinal herbs. For container gardening, use three separate large pots. As you dig deeper into growing food, you can start to utilize some permaculture principles. When you have a design in mind, you can start integrating companion planting, matching light and water requirements, rotating plantings in your garden and integrating beneficial insects. But to get started, herbs are an easy and forgiving choice for beginners.

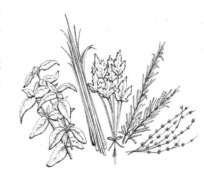

Try to grow herbs that you already buy (fresh or dried), such as basil, chives, rosemary, thyme, sage, oregano, parsley, dill and cilantro.

Herbs should be held in reverence and used with care. Herbs affect everyone differently and should therefore be used with caution. Common contraindications to the use of medicinal herbs include: pregnancy and lactation, heart disease, liver problems, chronic illnesses. Always consult a MD, ND or trained clinical herbalist before integrating herbs into your daily routine. In this book you will find very basic information on common herbs. For more detailed information on herbs consult books by Rosemary Gladstar.

Culinary herbs are highly medicinal. They serve a dual purpose and therefore, are incredibly important to have around. I like to stock up on culinary herbs throughout the season, typically dry or dehydrate them and combine in a Mason jar. My favorite combination is a blend of thyme, oregano, sage, basil, savory, mint, lemon balm, echinacea root, chamomile and dandelion leaves. I brew them throughout the winter to boost our immune systems and to aid in the relief of cold and flu symptoms. Some culinary herbs improve respiratory function, purify the blood, cleanse the liver and kidneys, and relieve stomach upsets. They may contain antibacterial and antiviral properties, as well as immune-building properties.

Herbs are either perennial, annual or biennial. Perennial plants return year after year. Annuals complete their life cycle within one year. Biennials return one year and go dormant for the next, alternating growing cycles. Do your research and make a handy chart of all your plants, including seeding recommendations, spacing and light requirements. It is best to buy perennial plant starts (preferably organic) from a local nursery. I sow tender annuals in trays for transplanting and sow hardy annuals directly into the ground.

Below is a list of some favorite culinary herbs to grow in your kitchen window, in containers or in your yard.

Annuals

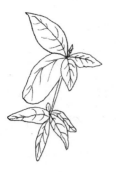

Basil (Annual/Full sun/Likes warm weather/Prefers well-drained and moist soil)

Culinary uses: Basil is known for its unique flavor and for being crushed into pesto. It makes a wonderful addition to pasta sauces, sandwiches, salads and many Italian dishes. Purple basil can be crushed into delicious pink lemonade. Lemon basil can be used to flavor fish or poultry. Cinnamon basil makes a delicious tea, as does holy basil (tulsi), which is considered a sacred herb in many religions.

Medicinal uses: Basil has strong antibacterial and antioxidant properties that help alleviate indigestion, cold and flu symptoms, asthma and bronchitis. It is also high in magnesium and helps to improve blood flow.

A plethora of varieties can be grown from seed or transplanted from a plant start. Some well-known varieties include purple basil, lemon basil and cinnamon basil.

Cilantro (Annual/Full sun/Likes cool or mild weather/ Prefers well-drained soil)

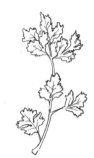

Culinary uses: Cilantro is notorious for its love-it-or–hate-it reputation but has been used in many global cuisines.

Medicinal uses: Cilantro aids in digestion, eases menstrual cramps and helps to relieve colic in infants when the breastfeeding mother drinks cilantro tea.

Dill (Annual/Full sun/Likes cooler weather/Prefers well-drained soil)

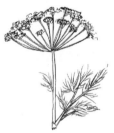

Culinary uses: Dill, a natural salt substitute, is known for its unique slightly salty addition to pickled cucumbers.

Medicinal uses: Dill aids in digestion, is soothing for anxiety and is rich in mineral salts.

Fennel (Annual/Full sun/Likes warm weather/Prefers well-drained moist soil)

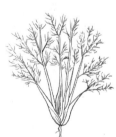

Culinary uses: Fennel, an aromatic herb, tastes like anise or licorice. The bulb can be chopped and tossed in olive oil and roasted with root vegetables. It is a nice addition to soups and salads.

Medicinal uses: Fennel has been used to treat anxiety and depression as well as digestive upsets and colic in babies.

Perennials

Lavender (Perennial or annual/Full sun/ Likes warm weather/Prefers sandy, well-drained soil)

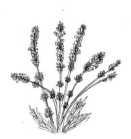

Some varieties are perennials. Check to see which variety grows best for your region.

Culinary uses: Lavender is the spotlight herb in Herbes de Provence, a popular blend containing savory, oregano, rosemary and thyme. Lavender has a sweet flowery flavor and makes a delightful addition to cookies, scones, granola or lemonades. Lavender lemon shortbread cookies are one of my favorites. Lavender honey lemonade is a refreshing summertime drink.

Medicinal uses: Lavender has a soothing effect on the body. It can be used to treat digestive upsets. It has antibacterial and antiviral properties and is rich in antioxidants.

Chives (Perennial/Full sun/Tolerates warm and cool weather/Prefers fertile soil that is moist and well-drained)

Culinary uses: Chives have a mild onion/garlic flavor and are an excellent addition to any savory meal. Its flowers are also edible. Chives are easily cut with kitchen scissors.

Medicinal uses: Chives have antioxidant properties and have been used in helping to lower cholesterol and blood pressure. They are high in vitamins A, C and K and rich in calcium and iron.

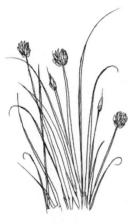

Garlic Chives, Aka Chinese leeks, (Perennial/Full sun/Tolerates warm and cool weather)

Culinary uses: Garlic chives have a robust garlic flavor and are also a wonderful addition to any savory dish. Their leaves are flat, like leeks, as opposed to those of standard chives, which are hollow and tubular.

Lemon Balm (Perennial/Full sun/Likes warm weather/Prefers moist and fertile soil)

Culinary uses: Use lemon balm fresh in salads. Cut thin strips with scissors and use to garnish fish. Make a delicious lemon balm tea or elixir. Lemon balm cordial is delicate and tasty. Cordial is a syrupy liquor made from a sugar or honey infused with concentrated herb tea.

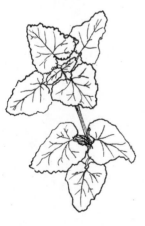

Medicinal uses: For centuries, lemon balm has been called the vitality herb and has been used to treat ailments including anxiety, cold and flu symptoms, fever, digestive complaints, headaches and insomnia. It can also act as a natural insect repellent; crush a handful of leaves and rub on exposed skin.

Lovage (Perennial/Full sun/Tolerates warm and cool weather/Prefers moist soil)

Culinary uses: Lovage, also called cutting celery, has a strong and crisp celery-like flavor. Fresh or dried, it makes a lovely addition to soups, stews and casseroles.

Medicinal uses: Lovage has been used to treat headaches, digestive upsets and fatigue.

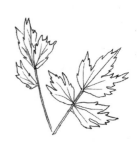

Mint (Perennial/Full sun or partial shade/Likes warm weather/Will thrive in various soil conditions)

Culinary uses: Mint makes a wonderful fresh addition to Thai and Vietnamese dishes, as well as fruit salads and ice cream. Mint and yogurt are a surprisingly delicious combination, found in Mediterranean cucumber salads. It can also be used in many beverages like lemonade and various cocktails.

Medicinal uses: Mint has a cooling effect on the body. It is great for the digestive system and helps reduce fevers. Mint tea is a soothing gargle for sore throats.

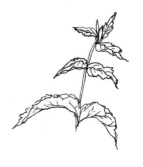

Oregano (Perennial/Full sun/Likes warmer weather/ Prefers well-drained soil)

Culinary uses: Oregano, known for its potent flavor in Mediterranean foods, has actually been used worldwide for centuries. Its zesty flavor complements soups, stews, sauces, beans and rice.

Medicinal uses: Oregano has antibiotic, antibacterial and antifungal properties. Tea made from fresh or dried oregano aids in digestion and relieves menstrual cramps, coughs and colds.

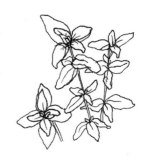

Parsley (Biannual/Full sun/Tolerates warm and cool weather/Prefers moist, well- drained soil)

Culinary uses: Parsley, a wonderfully flavorful garnish, also makes a fresh and delicious addition to any savory dish. The two primary types are curled and flat-leaf. It is the key ingredient in taboulei, a Middle Eastern salad. Use parsley fresh in salads or add it to green smoothies.

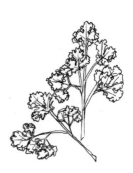

Medicinal uses: Parsley is among the most medicinal of the culinary herbs. It is high in iron, calcium and vitamins K, A, C and B. It is rich in antioxidants, has anticancer properties and helps strengthen the immune system. It can aid in digestion and offer relief for colds and flu.

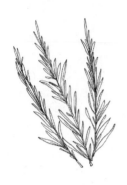

Rosemary (Tender perennial in northern climates/Full sun/Likes warm weather/Needs well-drained soil)

Culinary uses: Rosemary pairs well with root vegetables, such as potatoes and turnips, and bread.

Medicinal uses: Rosemary is a nutrient-rich herb containing many phytonutrients as well as iron, potassium and calcium. It is high in vitamins A and C and exhibits antioxidant, antibacterial and anti-inflammatory properties. It has been used to treat depression and headaches, as well as cold and flu symptoms.

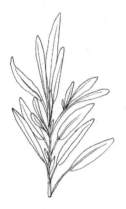

Sage (Hardy perennial/Full sun/Likes warmer weather/Prefers light, well-drained soil)

Culinary uses: Sage, most commonly used in stuffing, is a delicious addition to savory dishes including soups and hearty stews. Pan-fried, sage turns crispy and silvery and makes a great addition to pastas or butternut squash bisque.

Medicinal uses: Sage has a long history as a highly revered medicinal herb. This tonic herb can be used to treat colds, flu viruses, fevers and sore throats. First Nations have used it for centuries as a smudging and clearing herb.

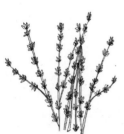

Thyme (Perennial/Full sun/Likes warm weather/Prefers well-drained soil)

Thyme, one of the most cold-hardy herbs, will be found alive and well under a layer of ice in the garden.

Culinary uses: Thyme, one of my favorite herbs, has a rich spicy flavor that is excellent in soups, hearty stews, pasta dishes and breads.

Medicinal uses: Thyme is an antiseptic herb. It aids digestion, alleviates cold symptoms, clears congestion in the lungs, reduces fever, chills, aches and pains, and helps to eliminate toxins in the body. Drink a honey-sweetened tea steeped with fresh or dried thyme.

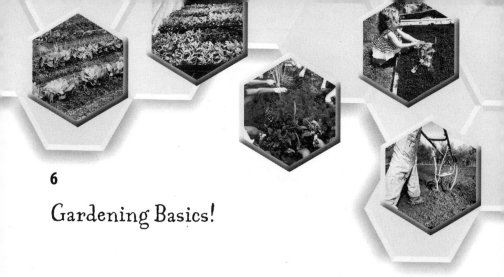

6

Gardening Basics!

A GOOD WAY TO EASE INTO GARDENING is to start with the landscape. Sustainable, native and edible landscaping are a few great methods to adopt to get your thumbs green.

Most folks prefer a freshly mowed lawn with pristine and neat landscaping. Unfortunately, most landscape companies are not practicing sustainable techniques. With billions of homes in the United States alone, non-sustainable yards can truly leave a negative carbon footprint. Pesticide and herbicide residue from lawn applications can be found not only in the soil, but also in the water supply and even the air long after their application. Overexposure to these chemicals has been linked to many life-threatening illnesses, including cancer.

Beautiful lawns can certainly be achieved sustainably. Remember that the idea of using chemicals to grow plants is a recent one and came from the ironically named Green Revolution. Transitioning to a more sustainable lawn is a wonderful way to make a green contribution to the future of the planet. Native landscaping attracts pollinators and will make a huge difference in your region's ecosystem.

Get out and be inspired by individuals who have taken a stance to avoid chemicals on their lawn and use sustainable landscaping methods. In my hometown in Missouri, Terry Winkleman founded a very cool project. The Sustainable Backyard Tour, a St. Louis organization that aims to showcase local sustainable backyards, sets an example for anyone wanting to go green. They focus on those who have replaced invasive and energy-intensive plants with native flowers, shrubs and trees. They have great ideas for backyard chicken coops, rainwater catchment systems, compost bins and other urban gardening projects. Visit sustainablebackyardtour .com.

Another of my favorite local companies is an inspirational model founded by Joseph Heller after he noticed "a need for sustainable landscape solutions in the St. Louis area." Simply Sustainable Landscaping, owned by Joseph and his wife, Brandy McClure-Heller, is solution-focused, based on individual needs and desires. Their landscaping services include native garden installation, small-scale prairie restoration, rain garden installation, edible landscaping, vegetable garden installation, and compost bin installation and education. They landscape with native plants, emphasizing perennial flowers, shrubs and trees instead of annuals; they follow organic practices, and they remove invasive plant species. Brandy focuses on artistic landscape design and integrating medicinal herbs and edibles into landscapes. In their collaborative creative process, Joe chooses the plant material and draws a rough sketch of his vision, and Brandy brings the landscape to life in a beautiful artistic rendition. They enjoy creating gardens that are both aesthetically pleasing and functional. Visit simplysustainablelandscaping.com for some great landscaping ideas.

Their top ten favorite full-sun native plant varieties for the Midwest are Missouri evening primrose, rattlesnake master, compass plant, purple coneflower, Baptisia, Eastern blazing star, prickly pear, smooth hydrangea, white fringe tree and bur oak. Their top ten favorite shade-loving plant varieties are Virginia bluebells, trillium, May apple, Solomon's seal, columbine, Jacob's ladder, witch hazel, flowering dogwood, sassafras and pawpaw.

Edible landscaping incorporates fruits and vegetables into the environment in an aesthetically pleasing way, bringing sustainability and functionality to life. Landscapers choose the perfect fruits and vegetables for full sun, partial sun and shady spots throughout a yard and arrange them in a functional and creative way.

Sustainable landscape designers and architects are changing the world one lawn at a time. Be inspired by the artists, environmentalists and plant lovers who make this profession their passion. In this vast field, practitioners focus on different features, from edible landscaping to native/heritage gardens to pollination gardens and more. You can incorporate the basic principles of good landscape design into your own home projects, as well as call upon these professionals for help.

Gardening for Beginners: Planting Your First Garden

Everyone is capable of growing their own food and medicine.

Seed soil water sun weed harvest share repeat ... Growing can be as simple as you need it to be.

So many people are intimidated by gardening, but it can be simple, fun and highly rewarding. I recommend you start planting the things that you love to eat or that you find beautiful.

Chances are your passion for gardening will grow with each changing season. You can start a balcony container garden or a small backyard garden for less than 20 dollars.

Embrace organic!

Gardening Step One: Determining Your Zone and Soil Type

The first steps are to determine which planting zone you reside in and the type of soil you have in the location you wish to grow a garden. The plant hardiness zone map helps to determine which plants will thrive in your area. Zones are determined by day length, soil temperatures, climate, air temperatures and first and last frost dates. Growing periods vary around the globe. What may be blooming in spring in your backyard at a specific time may still be dormant in other parts of the country or vice versa. Search for your specific region's plant hardiness zone at planthardiness.ars.usda.gov. Regional zone maps are accessible through local university extension offices.

For example, tomatoes thrive in hot temperatures while greens thrive in cooler temperatures. However, there are plenty of loopholes in gardening. For instance, you can find the time of the year that mimics the place of origin of a particular plant. There are specific times indicated by soil temperature when certain plants thrive. This will vary from zone to zone. For instance, Mediterranean herbs thrive in Midwest summers. Plants that wouldn't typically grow in a cooler climate can grow inside a temperature-regulated high tunnel or greenhouse.

It will also be beneficial to determine where your garden will be (or already is) located and to make notes about its microclimate. Write down where it is sunny, shady, windy, etc. Note also whether a plant will be grown on an incline. Making and keeping diagrams and drawings of your garden is very helpful!

Some plants grow well by directly sowing them into the ground, such as root vegetables and greens. Others do best when seeds are planted into small containers or a seed tray with several cells indoors under grow lights or in a greenhouse so that roots are well-established before being transplanted outdoors. For example, carrot seeds thrive when planted directly into the ground whereas tomatoes do best when transplanted.

To determine your soil type, you can go the precision route and get a soil test through your local extension office. This analysis helps to determine the biochemistry of the soil. The amount of different minerals and nutrients in your soil indicates which plants will thrive in that specific soil structure. The analysis also allows you to compare the ideal nutrient levels to those present in your specific soil. Typically, the test will come with suggestions about how to best improve your soil composition.

For a less complicated route, use a pitchfork or a shovel to turn over the soil in a section where you want your garden to be. Is your soil hard clay or mud? Is it loose and loamy? Is it sandy or rocky? Look around your yard and note which plants are already thriving. Clay soil and sandy soil benefit from the addition of compost. Good growing soil has a variety of organic materials and aggregates; it is loose and loamy, and the humus (organic material formed from decomposition of plant and animal matter) is dark in color.

Gardening Step Two: Choosing Seeds Based on Your Zone and Soil Types

Seed selection is an important part of planning your garden, yet many beginning gardeners feel intimidated by this process. Seed selection is more than just thumbing through seed catalogs and choosing the most eye-catching varieties. There are factors to consider such as heat resistance, drought tolerance, disease resistance and the climate that the specific variety thrives in. You can check with local farmers, gardeners or extension office for help choosing varieties that do well in your region. There is no sense in reinventing the wheel. Follow these simple steps to ensure a stress-free seed selection process!

1. Make a list of your favorite fruits and vegetables. It is important to grow what you love to eat, so that the harvest will not go to waste. If you like, you can also plan to donate and share your harvest with friends, family members, neighbors and community food banks.

2. Determine whether or not your favorites will grow in your specific growing zone. From here, cull a modified list of seeds that you will want to obtain for your garden.

3. Determine the specific growing requirements for your chosen plants, including light, spacing and water. Make sure to record this information in an easily accessible location such as a gardening journal or a paper taped to your refrigerator. Not only will writing it down help you remember and learn about these plants, it will also be a useful resource for all future gardening adventures.

4. Every plant has many different varieties. Choose seed varieties that are specific to your needs. Some varieties are labeled as drought resistant, disease resistant, etc.

5. Once you have your varieties narrowed down, order the seeds through a reputable company that signs a non-GMO pledge such as Seeds of Change, Johnny's Selected Seeds, Baker Creek Heirloom Seeds, The Rare Vegetable Seed Consortium, Seed Savers Exchange, Seed Geeks or Morgan County Seeds. You may also visit a local nursery and consult the staff; they are often eager and excited to help.

6. Select new and unique varieties as well as heirloom seeds. Try something new each time you buy seeds. You will be amazed at the incredible and beautiful variety within a single species of plant! We love to grow beautiful and unique specialty produce, and don't believe anyone should feel limited by conventional varieties of plants.

Beginner's Guide to Seasonal Organic Vegetable Gardening (from a Midwestern Perspective)

Winter

The winter is a great time to start planning your garden and ordering seeds. Seedsofchange.com has an excellent variety of organic seeds. Rareseeds.com (Baker Creek Heirloom Seeds) is a great resource for heirloom seeds.

Organize your seeds according to planting dates. For small-scale gardening, accordion-style organizers work well.

Start the following seeds indoors under grow lights or in a greenhouse mid-February through mid-April: broccoli, bok choi, kohlrabi, cabbage, onions, scallions, eggplant, early tomatoes and peppers.

Plan the layout of your garden. Sketch where you want each crop to go. Keep in mind companion planting, light and water requirements, height, spacing and aesthetics. There are a number of books available at your local library on vegetable gardening that offer garden plans ranging from raised beds to acre plantings.

Early Spring (When the Ground Thaws, Typically Early March)

If you have a large garden that gets plenty of sun, prepare your space as soon as the ground is ready. The ground should be thawed and slightly dry. Use a broad fork or a potato fork to turn the top layer of soil over and gently break it up. Your goal should be a fine tilth soil. Be sure to add plenty of compost, bags of leaves, grass clippings and green manure before you prep. These soil additions will feed your plants throughout the year.

You can easily create raised beds with straw bales, cinder blocks and un-treated scrap wood or heat-treated pallets. In a raised bed, additions of any of the following layers would help create good living soil and provide organic pathways for roots: leaves, followed by straw, grass clippings, more leaves and compost. Next, add half compost and half topsoil. Finally, your top layer should be well-decomposed compost mixed with topsoil. You want your top layer to have a fine tilth so that it is easy to sow seeds.

Spring

After the last frost when the ground can be worked, plant the following from seed directly into the ground: spinach, carrots, peas, chard, kale, salad mix, lettuce, radishes, beets and turnips. You may purchase established vegetable plants (that you were not able to plant from seed in late winter or early spring) and transplant them into your garden. Nurseries carry a variety of plants for vegetable gardening. Plant comfrey near your beds as it is a natural fertilizer. Cut leaves added to garden beds as mulch will give your beds extra nutrition.

Weed regularly. For young seedlings, be sure to keep the soil weed-free with hand tools. It's a good idea to lightly weed your garden by hand often rather than try to do it all at once; weeding on a regular basis will save you time in the long run and will improve the quality of your garden.

For transplants, the use of weed barriers such as weed cloths, sheet mulching, straw and compost are important for suppressing weeds and re-taining moisture.

Use soaker hoses to keep your seed beds well-watered until they sprout. Water on a regular basis once plants are established, though water needs vary from plant to plant.

Late Spring

Tomatoes, winter squash, summer squash, cucumbers, melons, peppers, beans, okra, raspberries, blackberries and herbs such as basil and dill can be planted to enjoy in the summer. Plant them from seed in your prepared garden beds or from transplants. Plant potatoes from seed and sweet potato slips.

Summer

In the summer, plant the same crops you planted in early spring. You can repeat the process with warm-season crops and then again for fall crops. Just follow a planting guide for your zone or region.

Fall

Plant carrots and greens to overwinter and enjoy the next spring. Harvest everything from your garden before the first frost. Clear out your garden beds and cover them with cardboard, tarps or landscape fabric.

Start a Basic Backyard Garden for 50 dollars (10×10-foot Plot)

The wonderful thing about gardening is that it can be done simply by collectively gathering resources and sharing the end harvest.

This guide factors in the kindness of neighbors, the generosity of friends and relatives, and the resourcefulness of the gardener's mindset. With 50 dollars and some creativity, you can create a basic garden in your backyard using the minimum number of new tools and resources. Not only are you saving money, but you are promoting the use of recycled materials. Starting a garden bed can be done during any season. If you want to have a bed prepared for spring, however, it is best to start just after the ground thaws. Throughout the world, gung-ho gardeners always find a way to grow food, despite the season. Check with your friends and neighbors. See what seeds they are sowing when you get started. The barter system is tremendously helpful for gardening. Sharing resources is one of the best ways to approach life in general, I've found!

First, gather your resources. In our estimation, these are the only things you'll need to buy.

* Seeds and plants: 30 dollars. Seed packets average about 2 dollars each or you can save your own. Neighbors and friends can go in on bulk seed orders to save money. Plants average 3 dollars each. Smaller nurseries tend to have better prices.
* Garden fork: 5 dollars. You can find a used garden fork in decent condition from friends, flea markets, Craigslist or Freecycle networks. A garden fork is heavy duty and has four long tines, typically forged from a solid piece of carbon steel, making it great for turning over compacted soil. If you can't find one to buy in your budget, borrow one.
* Compost: 6 dollars per bag or free from a friend or farmer. Most cities have a free compost program.
* Straw bale: 3 dollars. Check Craigslist under "farm and garden" or ask a local farmer. Straw bales can often be purchased at farm or seed stores.
* Garden hose. Most folks already own a garden hose. Neighbors might have an extra you can borrow in exchange for a few homegrown vegetables.

If you have a higher budget, consider investing in a broad fork, a tool that loosens and aerates the soil without disturbing the living network of micro-organisms, bacteria and fungi.

Now, stock up on these free and repurposed useful supplies.

* Perennial (native) plants to attract pollinators: Free from friend or neighbors
* Vessels for starting seeds. These make excellent seed-starting containers and can be saved throughout the winter to start seeds in the spring: coffee bags, toilet paper rolls, water bottles, recycled plastic quart containers, reused milk cartons, egg cartons.
* Plant labels made from recycled materials (use permanent marker, crayons or waxed pencils to label): Old venetian blinds (simply cut individual blinds to the desired size), recycled yogurt containers cut into strips, reused popsicle sticks
* Soil: Some city parks have a free soil program. A park may offer the following soil options:
  * Fill dirt: Good for a base layer or filler, but the nutrient level is unpredictable
  * Topsoil: Generally the top two inches of soil, which is more nutrient-rich and brings your garden soil up to a more balanced and preferred level of nutrients to benefit the plants
  * Compost: A combination of various detritus materials with a soil base that includes mostly yard waste, such as leaves, grass clippings, small branches and twigs
  * Chip mulch: Shredded limbs and trunks of trees are good for pathways, mulching around trees and perennial natives, shrubs and flower and herb beds. Its job is to protect roots and maintain moisture levels. If you dump and spread chip mulch in your future garden bed and let it rest for one year, it not only will smother the weeds but also will break down into more of a loamy humus layer, making it an excellent foundation for permaculture garden beds or edible landscapes.
  * Sand: Very useful especially when mixed with compost for growing herbs. Sand is also a good additive for fast drainage. It also works well mixed with compost for starting seeds to promote better drainage, as a top dressing or as mulch for heating up the soil around the base of herb plants.
* Free mulch for garden beds:
  * Black and white newspaper (no color or glossy ink)

- Leaves or leaf litter from your yard or neighbors'
- Grass clippings
- Weeds (as you weed your garden, lay the pulled weeds down flat around each plant to act both as green manure and to also help suppress the growth of more weeds)
- Burlap coffee bags

Now, you're ready to prepare your garden spot.

1. In an area of your front or backyard, find a somewhat level spot that gets full sun for at least six hours per day. Mark out a 10-by-10-foot plot using a few stones or pieces of scrap wood.

2. Two weeks before you turn under the area for your garden, spray a mixture of one part vinegar (white vinegar is the cheapest) to two parts water on this plot. This will act as a prevention measure for managing weeds as well as insects.

3. After your plot has sat for two weeks, it is time to start digging. With your foot, press a potato fork halfway into the ground, using leverage to turn under the soil. Once all of the soil in the plot is turned up, use the potato fork to break up large clumps of soil.

4. Let the plot sit for a day or two so that the weeds die back. Use the fork again to break up the soil to create a finer dirt.

5. Spread a bag (or wheelbarrow full) of compost over the plot. Work the compost into the soil until an even consistency is achieved.

6. Plant your garden with season-appropriate seeds or plant starts. For instance, greens do well in cooler weather, and tomatoes do well in hot weather. Mulch established plants with straw or whatever mulch you have on hand.

Building Raised Beds

Simple raised beds can be built using pallets, which are typically free. Local businesses such as warehouses and shipping facilities with pallets out back are glad to give them away because it often saves them money. But it is best to ask the business owner directly for permission. Get the ones labeled HT, which means they have been heat-treated.

Sketch out your garden design and, over the course of a few weeks, start building simple raised beds with scrap wood or pallets, a hammer and some weatherproof nails. If you are a carpenter, more elaborate beds can be built.

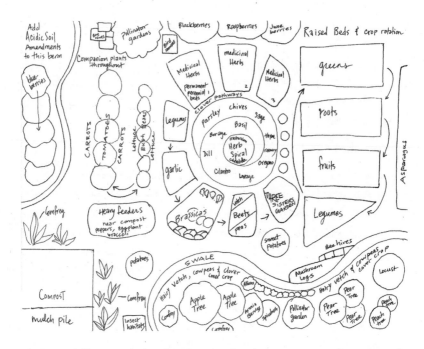

Fill the bed frame with equal parts topsoil and compost. See Chapter Six for instructions on how to build a raised bed using pallets. *Gaia's Garden* by Toby Hemenway offers design ideas for home gardeners.

Building Your Compost System

Shipping pallets can also be used to quickly build an inexpensive compost system. There are so many benefits to composting that I can't even mention them all here! At its most basic, composting in your home allows you to make your own healthy soil, feed nutrients to your crops and reduce waste in your household.

A pallet compost system is very easy. Refer to Chapter Four for how to build your own compost bin system.

Basic Materials for Gardening

* Terra cotta pots and wooden planters, your best options for container gardening
* River rocks, loose gravel or sand to line the bottom of your pots for adequate drainage
* Nutrient-rich potting soil. We get ours through a great company called Beautiful Land Products.

* Watering can or hose
* Compost (broken down, of course). While your compost system is developing, you can buy compost or borrow from a friend or neighbor.
* Patience and a little time to weed and water your plants. Think of it as your daily meditation hour. Try to take this one hour to connect to the world around you and turn off your electronic devices. This hour can be used to ground yourself, to focus on your breath, to dedicate energy to making your plant friends thrive.

Instinct gardening also has the tendency to work surprisingly well. Decisions are made by trusting your intuition. For example, if you are wondering about spacing requirements for cabbage, simply imagine the standard size of a cabbage, adding a few inches on either side for leaves. Gauge the spacing based on how large the end product is.

I suggest keeping a journal to record the steps you take as you become a full-fledged grower. You might say, "I don't need a journal, I will remember this," but I assure you, growing can develop into a slight addiction, and you will soon find yourself with a tiny jungle on your balcony. Based on my experience, I have found that certain small details seem to meld into one another over time, so keeping a record of your green thumb adventures can help you out year after year.

Connect with Others Through Gardening

* Get excited about gardening!
* Join your local garden club.
* Start your own gardening club.
* Check out local gardening and farming meet-ups online.
* Host gardening parties in your yard and the yards of your plant enthusiast friends.
* Offer to start a community garden in your neighborhood or community.
* Getting friends and family involved to help lighten the workload can bring excitement and joy to any gardening project.

A Garden Oasis!

Most importantly, transform your yard into a garden oasis! Turn your backyard garden into a place where you can retreat to and relax, a place where you grow fruits, vegetables and herbs that you love and will use or share and that bring you fulfillment and happiness.

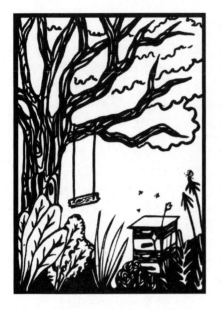

Imagine yourself in the spring in a warm and sunlit area of your yard, planting your own vegetable garden. You could be providing fresh organically grown produce for your friends and family for an entire growing season. The benefits of organic gardening are remarkable:

* You will know exactly how your food is being grown without worrying about unsafe pesticides.
* Freshly picked organic vegetables provide an excellent source of vitamins, minerals and nutrients to your diet. Their taste is fresh, crisp and delightful. They are packed with authentic flavor and will improve your health.
* Growing your own produce cuts costs tremendously at the supermarket.
* The joy of witnessing the firsthand experience of the seed-to-table connection is immeasurable.

Natural Weed and Pest Management

Sheet mulching, also known as lasagna gardening, is a wonderful way to keep your garden bed weed-free. Sheet mulching is essentially layering compost, leaf mulch, grass clippings, newspaper, more compost and straw or mulch around each of your plants to help suppress weeds, add nutrients and retain moisture.

Companion planting is an excellent way to keep garden pests at bay. Inter-planting onions or hot peppers can help deter unwanted garden pests from susceptible crops. Find out which pests are most prevalent in your region and plant crops that will deter them. Companion planting is also a great way to add healthy diversity to your garden. Borage and marigolds help attract pollinators while deterring unwanted pests from the garden.

Cover cropping is the process of growing a crop to feed the soil. The following can be planted and then incorporated into your soil to add nutrients to the soil: legumes, cow peas, hairy vetch, winter wheat, sunflowers.

Row covers (weed barriers) are usually a white airy material used to create a physical barrier from swarms of insects and migrating birds. They also help to protect crops from frost and can be used to slightly extend the growing season.

Hand picking and eliminating soft-bodied insects such as cabbage loopers and horn worms might be necessary. If the problem is too intense, it may just be best to remove that plant from your garden altogether. Place the plant in a bucket of vinegar water to prevent the insect from going to your neighbors' crops or feed to your chickens.

Natural sprays such as PyGanic and Dipel can be effective, but they are expensive. Homemade sprays can be made in the blender (use an extension cord to make this outside!). Goggles, gloves and masks must be used when making, handling and applying potent natural pest sprays.

Combine ½ cup water, 4 raw onions (chopped), 10 whole cloves of garlic and 12 cayenne peppers in the blender and blend until smooth. Strain mixture into a colander inside a large pot. Line the colander with cheesecloth. Dilute with 1 gallon of water. Pour strained mixture into a backpack sprayer or into small spray bottles. Be sure to label clearly and keep out of the reach of children. Apply to crops to prevent pests or to treat plants that have harmful insects on them.

Crop rotation should be done after harvesting each crop each season. The soil needs a break from heavy feeders such as peppers as well as a variance in root depth. Additionally, crop rotation limits insect and pest problems.

Pollinator gardens are essential to every healthy garden system. Without pollinators, our plates would be empty. Every vegetable garden should integrate plants and flowers that attract pollinators such as honeybees and butterflies as well as ladybugs and other beneficial insects. Native flowers from your region are the best to attract pollinators. However, companion plants such as borage, calendula and marigolds serve a dual purpose: they attract pollinators and keep harmful pests away from your crops. Bright, showy, colorful flowers such as zinnias also attract pollinators.

By following these steps, you will acquire a green thumb in no time and will be enjoying a lovely garden and a bountiful harvest of fresh, homegrown, seasonal, organic produce this summer and fall. Avid vegetable gardeners are able to enjoy the fruits of their labor year-round with careful planning and maintenance, and over time, you will too!

Additional Tips for Harvesting and Storing Produce

* Use practical knowledge when determining ideal conditions for harvesting specific crops. Use proper techniques for each specific crop, which can be found online or in gardening books.

* Harvest greens with a sharp knife early in the morning before the sun shines directly on them. Place them in a cool water bath and spin them directly after harvest.
* Tomatoes are best harvested once the dew lifts in the afternoon.
* Think about plant health when harvesting. For instance, only use a small paring knife to harvest summer squash. A large knife may damage the entire plant, attracting squash bugs and making the plant vulnerable to diseases.
* Keep harvested produce in cool shaded areas and use a cool water bath to revive and retain freshness.
* When displaying produce for purchase, it is best to present it as though it were being displayed at a grocer. Wash produce well, have consistent bunches, remove yellow leaves and don't include blemished produce.
* Root crops store best with a layer of field dirt left on them; wash just before use. Root crops may be stored in sand in a cool dark space to preserve longevity.

More Fun for Your Garden

Now that we have the basics covered ... here are some beautiful additions to your garden!

Specialty Crops

Specialty crops are typically fairly easy to grow. Specialty crops usually include a long list of fruits, vegetables, herbs and edible flowers that are not readily available in a given area. Chefs are especially drawn to using specialty crops in their culinary repertoire.

For example, Sun Gold cherry tomatoes are revered among chefs and market-goers for their vibrant color and superb sweet flavor. They are a non-GMO hybrid variety and are our favorite variety of cherry tomatoes. Kohlrabi, a beautiful cross between a cabbage and a turnip, is bred from wild cabbage and originated in northern Europe around 500 years ago. The flavor of kohlrabi is similar to that of broccoli stems. Enjoy kohlrabi raw, steamed, sautéed or roasted. Raw is best as kohlrabi is rich in protein and vitamin C and is an excellent source of dietary fiber.

Edible Flowers

My favorite edible flowers are nasturtiums, which have a spicy zing to them. They are gorgeous topped on cupcakes. I decorated my wedding cake with nasturtiums and calendula flowers. They come in vibrant colors including red, yellow, orange and peach.

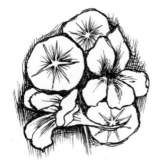

Violets are also among my favorites. They are a striking purple color and are so dainty and beautiful.

Chefs and foodies alike love to incorporate edible flowers into their dishes. Smaller flowers make beautiful garnishes, while the larger flowers can be candied or stuffed.

My favorite edible flowers include anise hyssop, apple blossoms, basil flowers, black locust flowers, borage, calendula, chamomile, chervil flowers, chicory, chives, chrysanthemum, coriander flower, crabapple blossoms, dandelion, dianthus, dill flowers, day

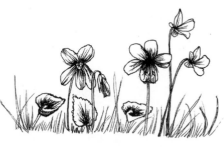

lilies, English daisy, fennel flowers, garden pea flowers, garden sage flowers, grape hyacinth, hibiscus (rose of China and rose of Sharon), lavender, lemon balm flowers, lemon blossoms, marigolds (pot marigold, African marigold and signet marigold), marjoram flowers, mustard flowers, okra flowers, orange blossoms, oregano flowers, pansies, pineapple sage flowers, plum blossoms, radish flowers, redbud, red clover, rose petals, rosemary flowers, scarlet runner beans, scented geraniums, squash blossoms, summer savory flowers, thyme flowers, winter savory flowers and yucca flowers.

Heirloom Plants

Chefs and plant enthusiasts are also crazy about heirloom fruits and vegetables. These traditional or heritage plant varieties are preserved generation after generation through small-scale agricultural practice, saving the seed of their best crops year after year. They have not been genetically altered except by conscious selection. Some people will argue this is a form of genetic modification, albeit a "natural" form. Heirlooms generally have maintained their unique characteristics through open pollination. They are something to be cherished and protected, similar to a vintage heirloom pocket watch that a grandfather might pass down to his grandson. Small-scale family farmers and gardeners take pride in preserving plant heritage through seed saving.

Preserving heirloom plants is vital to the future of safe food. According to a report issued by the ETC Group revealing the monopolization of major industries, "The top 10 multinational seed companies now control 73 percent of the world's commercial seed market, up from 37 percent in 1995. The world's 10 biggest pesticide firms now control a whopping 90 percent of the global 44 billion dollar pesticide market. 10 companies control 76 percent of animal pharmaceutical sales. 10 animal feed companies control 52 percent of the global animal feed market."

Fortunately, there are many food revolutionaries who advocate for heirloom seed preservation. Jere Gettle, founder of Baker Creek Heirloom Seeds, named by the *New York Times* as "The Indiana Jones of Seeds," joins others from the grassroots up, working toward preservation of our incredible biodiversity. Joseph Simcox, the "Botanical Explorer," travels around the world collecting seeds from rare plants with the goal of preserving species. He founded the Gardens Across America Project, which provides free heirloom or highly rare seeds to gardeners with the intention of receiving 50 percent of their harvested seed to build a large rare vegetable seed consortium with his brother and sister, Patrick and Susan Simcox (explorewithjoseph .com). Rare and beautiful seeds from all over the world can be purchased at growrareseeds.com.

We can all do our part in our own gardens by saving our seeds and growing them year after year, sharing our harvests and sharing our seeds with our neighbors. Seed saving is one of the most important things a backyard organic gardener can do to preserve plant diversity.

One beautiful variety of beets is called the Chioggia beet, a pre-1840 Italian heirloom named after a fishing village. Beets are in the same family as chard and are native to Europe and the Mediterranean. Purple Beauty peppers, another stunning heirloom variety, have a gorgeous dark purple skin contrasted by lime green flesh and are said to have originated in Central and South America. They are sweet and delicious. Peppers are in the nightshade family, Solanaceae. Be careful, though. Because of cross-pollination, some peppers may be spicy.

Once you grow these unique beauties in your own garden, I'm sure you will enjoy them as much as we do. For years, my husband and I have been ordering seeds from Baker Creek Heirloom Seed Company. They have an amazing variety of heirloom seeds that produce some of the most vibrant and gorgeous fruits and vegetables that we have ever seen. Our all-time favorites, which we grow every year, include marketmore cucumber, green zebra tomato, Cherokee purple tomato, purple beauty peppers, red meat radish, Chioggia beets and golden beets.

Seed Saving

Late summer through late fall is a great time to save your own seeds. We like to use egg cartons and coffee filters. Lay your seeds in a single layer on coffee filters. Be sure to label them. You may think you will remember, but it is always good practice to label everything. When they are dry, you can sort and store them in labeled egg cartons or baby food jars. Be sure to put them in a mouse-proof area.

Seed saving is one of the most exciting and rewarding gardening processes. Just think: one pepper contains over 100 tiny seeds, each with the potential to become a plant that will produce nearly 100 peppers that each contain over 100 seeds. The process could go on forever. In pure form, seed saving represents the cycle of life and acts as a reminder of our humble beginnings.

It is important that gardeners learn how to save their own seeds. Organic seed prices have nearly doubled in the last ten years, and heirloom seed varieties can be difficult to find. We try to save as much seed as possible. In general, saved seeds should be used within one to three years, but I have had good luck planting some varieties of flowers with seed saved over five years earlier.

A Few Useful Tips on Seed Saving

My husband and I attended a workshop presented by Art Davidson, a knowledgeable and outgoing representative of Baker Creek Heirloom Seeds. He began with a simple question: "Why heirloom?" He followed that with a powerful answer, despite its simplicity: "Seeds are something worth saving, worth protecting." "You can't eat gold," he repeated throughout the talk. This really struck a chord with me. Ultimately, food, water, shelter and love are our most valuable resources and should be treated as gold.

There are many creative ways to save seeds. The internet is a great resource for how-to videos on seed saving. The online Baker Creek Catalog also has an excellent article. Whether you are just saving seeds for your own garden or for the future, the various methods of seed saving are important for growers to learn.

The following are major takeaways from Art's talk about seed saving:

* Dry your seeds on a paper plate for home seed saving and label clearly. As mentioned above, you can also use coffee filters or egg cartons.

* Seeds saved at home store the longest when kept in Mylar packets inside of glass jars in the freezer. They also store well in a dry place at 50 degrees or cooler. Seed banks store theirs at 28 degrees or below in glass jars or vials in rooms with dim light and dry air.

* When saving seeds on a larger scale, screen with various sized mesh for various sized seeds. Simply brush the seeds in a waving motion. The mesh needs to be rough enough to get the seed chaff off. Use a bin or something similar to catch the seeds. For rinsing and drying, use a wooden frame with a nylon screen.

* Isolation chambers are necessary for preserving heritage in many plants. You can build your own affordable isolation chambers using wooden frames or PVC pipes and floating row covers weighted down with sandbags. More detailed instructions are online. Art mentioned that it takes between six and twenty plants, as well as a swarm of bumblebees or mason bees, to ensure good pollination.

Seed Saving at Home

We have been saving our own seeds at home for years using the paper bag method! You don't need fancy equipment, just time, patience, brown paper bags or coffee filters and a marker. We include a brief description of the veggie or fruit. Because of the scale of our operation, we are unable to use isolation chambers. Additionally, our labels often disappear. Nevertheless, you can take your best and most beautiful veggies and save their seed. They may not turn out true to their parent plant, but you will save on seeds the following year, and who knows, you could even produce a beautiful new variety and name it after your kids! For heirloom seeds true to their heritage, we always go through rareseeds.com. As a perk, they have one of the most beautiful seed catalogs we have ever seen. Each year, we wrap our holiday gifts using the lovely pages of last year's seed catalogs!

Seed Geeks is a great resource! Marc and Angela Adler founded the company from their desire to live more sustainably, reconnect with their food sources, and help others to do the same. They strive to educate the community on the benefit and necessary preservation of heirloom seeds, seed saving and organic gardening. Visit www.seedgeeks.com to purchase heirloom open-pollinated seeds.

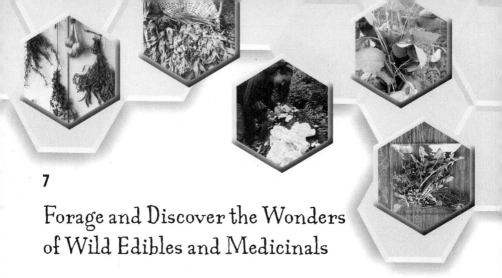

7

Forage and Discover the Wonders of Wild Edibles and Medicinals

W HILE YOU ANTICIPATE the farm fresh bounty, delve into the beautiful art of wild harvesting! It is fun to search for wild edibles in areas that are not sprayed with pesticides (another reason not to use chemical pesticides or herbicides). If you don't use chemicals on your lawn, you can harvest young, tender edible weeds from your own backyard. One of my greatest mentors is Penny Clark of Goods from the Woods. She created a business based on foraging seasonal and locally sourced foraged goods. Her line of teas, hydrosols and other natural products can be purchased at www. pinenut.com

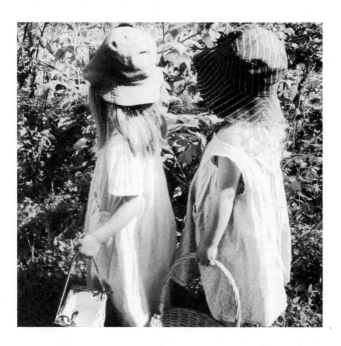

My dear friend and mentor, herbalist Colleen Smith, once described medicinal weeds as "plants growing in our backyards oftentimes so close to our back door that they seem as though they are just begging to get inside and alleviate what ails us." Herbalists across the globe are all aware of the powerful medicinal qualities of what most people refer to as "weeds." So many

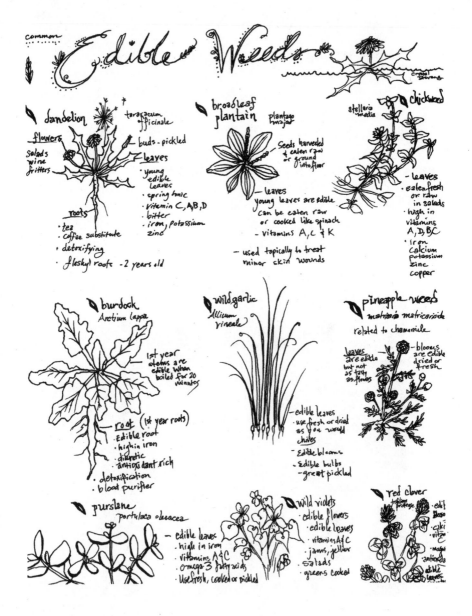

common

Edible Weeds

Crystal Stevens

dandelion
taraxacum officinale

flowers
Salads
wine
fritters

buds - pickled

leaves
· young edible leaves
· spring tonic
· Vitamin C, A B, D
· bitter
· iron, potassium
· zinc

roots
· tea
· Coffee substitute
· detoxifying
· fleshy roots - 2 years old

broadleaf plantain
plantago major

Seeds harvested & eaten raw or ground into floor

leaves
young leaves are edible can be eaten raw or cooked like spinach
- vitamins A, C & K

— used topically to treat minor skin wounds

chickweed
stellaria media

· leaves
eaten fresh or raw in salads
· high in vitamins A, D B C
· Iron Calcium potassium Zinc copper

burdock
Arctium lappa

1st year stems are edible when boiled for 20 minutes

root (1st year roots)
· Edible root
· high in iron
· diuretic
· antioxidant rich
· detoxification
· blood purifier

wild garlic
Allium vineale

· edible leaves
· use fresh or dried as you would chives
· Edible blooms
· Edible bulbs
— great pickled

pineapple weed
matricaria matricarioide
related to chamomile

leaves are edible but not as tasty as flowers

- blooms are edible dried or fresh

purslane
portulaca oleracea

— edible leaves
· high in iron
· vitamins A & C
· omega 3 fatty acids
· Use fresh, cooked or pickled

wild violets
· edible flowers
· edible leaves
· vitamins A & C
· jams, jellies
· Salads
· greens cooked

red clover
trifolium pratense
· edible Blooms
· cake vita E
· Magne antioxida
· edible leaves

people go to great lengths to achieve perfectly manicured lawns. I do not. My motto is that if it's growing, invasive or not, every plant has a purpose, whether it be for pollination; erosion prevention; food for animals, insects and people; or just for the sake of photosynthesis. Ralph Waldo Emerson said, "A weed is just a plant whose virtues have not yet been discovered."

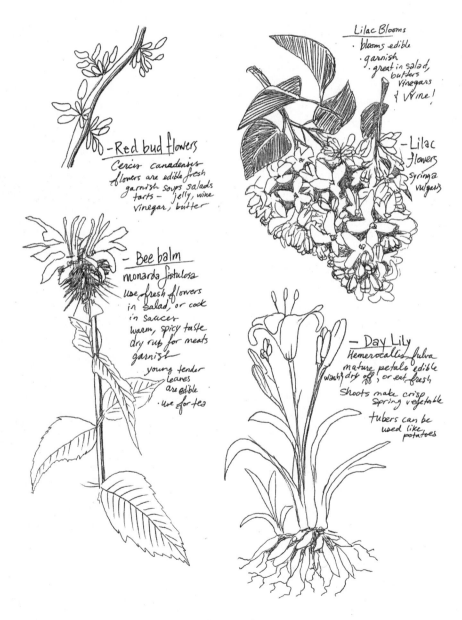

- Red bud flowers
Cercis canadensis
flowers are edible fresh
garnish soups salads
tarts - jelly, wine
vinegar, butter

Lilac Blooms
· blooms edible
· garnish
· great in salad,
butters
vinegars
& Wine!

- Lilac
flowers
syringa
vulgaris

- Bee balm
monarda fistulosa
use fresh flowers
in salad, or cook
in sauces
warm, spicy taste
dry rub for meats
garnish
young tender
leaves
are edible
· use for tea

- Day Lily
Hemerocallis fulva
mature petals edible
wash/dry off, or eat fresh
Shoots make crisp
spring vegetable
tubers can be
used like
potatoes

Wild Greens

In today's fast-paced world, it is hard not to lose our connection with nature and the understanding that we have an innate symbiotic relationship with plants and animals. We are inevitably responsible for the future of our planet. We are so busy with the reality and rituals of everyday life that we hardly notice the beauty beneath our feet, and even worse, we see what could ultimately heal us as something that is a nuisance. Serrated dandelions, soft and delicate red clovers, dainty wild onions and garlic, succulent chickweed and burly plantain are among the first to emerge, even before the grasses begin to green. They have all been dormant throughout the bitter cold winter and are ready to reach for the sun. The wild greens in spring are vibrant, and herbalists around the world consider them to be spring tonic plants.

Foraging for wild greens is one of our family's favorite pastimes, as well as a survival skill and lesson in character building that we enjoy teaching our children. They learn that weeds thrive in myriad growing conditions and under severe environmental stress, making them incredibly resilient and highly adaptable — like a dandelion growing through the cracks of concrete.

For centuries, weeds have been used worldwide for food and to treat ailments such as headaches, nausea, menstrual cramps, cold and flu symptoms, as well as labor and birth. Your local library should have a plethora of books on native plants and wild edibles specific to your region. Get creative and find recipes online or create your own.

Plant Identification

Identifying plants can be a very complex endeavor because many look alike, making them difficult to distinguish. Dandelion and plantain are easy to identify because they are everywhere. Plants look slightly different when growing in diverse conditions or throughout various stages of their life cycle. I have been an herbalist for over ten years, and it's still difficult for me to identify many plants. Taking someone's word on plant identification is only a good idea if they are a trained expert. When foraging, it is a good rule of thumb to harvest only a small amount — never take the entire stand of plants. Typically, it is a good idea to harvest only one quarter of what you find, if the plant population is abundant and thriving. Also, foragers should practice ethical harvesting by using appropriate techniques to remove plants.

Here are a few of my favorite edible weeds that grow in abundance in the Midwest and some throughout the United States.

Burdock root is edible and medicinal. Rich in calcium, potassium, copper, iron, chromium, flavonoid and vitamins, it is mucilaginous, meaning it coats the mucus membranes. Roots from young first-year burdocks can be harvested from early spring through late fall and cooked just like other root vegetables. It can be dehydrated and made into a detox tea or added to a coffee-substitute blend of dried roots that include dandelion and chicory.

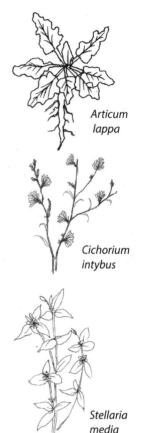

Articum lappa

Burdock root is excellent for detoxifying the liver, stimulating the appetite and aiding digestion. It has antifungal and antibacterial properties.

Chickweed is found in sunny and shady areas of most backyards. If you wild harvest chickweed, make sure the area is not sprayed with chemicals. It is high in vitamins C, A and B and packed with phytonutrients, magnesium, potassium, selenium, manganese and zinc.

Cichorium intybus

I enjoy taking nature walks with my children. They love to help me harvest chickweed because it is easy to pull! We bring it home, wash it and make a salad. I combine beeswax and an oil infused with chickweed, plantain, comfrey and dandelion for a salve that works well for cuts and scrapes.

Stellaria media

Dandelion has a plethora of medicinal uses. The roots are a powerful antioxidant and a friend to the digestive system. They can be roasted and used as a coffee substitute. The greens make an excellent pesto or salad and are high in vitamins and minerals. The flowers are high in iron, beta-carotene and vitamin C. Dandelion is a powerful detox herb. Aesthetically, the flowers make a nice garnish for any dish and are absolutely gorgeous in a refreshing herbal lemonade. Dandelion fritters are one of my favorite wild food dishes.

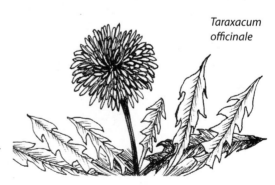

Taraxacum officinale

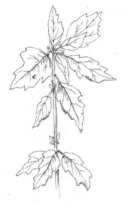

Chenopodium album

Lamb's quarters, also referred to as poor man's spinach, wild spinach or goosefoot, is found growing throughout the United States, maybe even in your own backyard. Just remember, as with any wild edible, be sure you identify it correctly before harvesting it. Use the leaves like spinach, cooked or raw in salads. Lamb's quarters is highly nutritious, packed with iron, vitamin C, calcium, riboflavin and niacin. We have been enjoying the lamb's quarters at La Vista since we began farming here. It actually contains trace elements of gold and silver, which is a natural antibiotic.

To clean lamb's quarters, immerse the whole plant and gently shake a few times. Add it to salads, smoothies, soups, stews, pastas, dough, cannelloni or lasagna.

Colleen Smith's Lamb's Quarters Pesto

    2 cups lamb's quarters leaves, stripped from their stalks (add
        other greens if needed)
    ½ cup extra virgin olive oil
    Pinch of salt
    ¼ cup toasted pine nuts (or nuts of your choice)
    Freshly grated Parmesan cheese (optional)

Blend all ingredients together in a food processor until smooth. For maximum nutrition, instead of olive oil, use ¼ cup apple cider vinegar and juice from half of a lemon and omit salt and cheese.

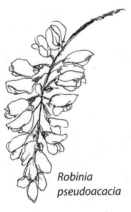

Robinia pseudoacacia

Black locust trees are native to Appalachia and thought to be invasive elsewhere in the US. The edible white and pink flowers have a high flavonoid content and a very pleasant fragrance. You can smell them in the Midwest from a few hundred feet away in May and early June. The flowers are sweet and have a lovely floral flavor. I love to make them into sweet dishes such as pastries or fritters with a honey yogurt dipping sauce. They can also be made into tea or wine. The rest of the tree is thought to be toxic.

Wild black raspberries have beautiful smooth (not ribbed) frosty bluish-purple thorny canes that poke out of the landscape in spring. Their serrated leaves, alternate and typically with one to three lobes, flush out in early summer, and the raspberries typically appear for a short period in mid-June. They are smaller, seedier and a little more tart than blackberries but make an excellent pie or jam.

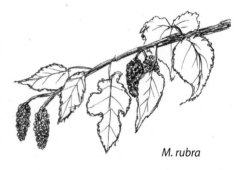

Rubus occidentalis

M. rubra

Mulberries: (Previously published in *Feast Magazine*) Ahh, the nostalgic feeling of collecting mulberries — fingers and lips stained a deep purple; the bittersweet flavor of the leaves just enough of a sweetness to keep picking more; the juicy mulberries bursting with flavor; their aroma reminiscent of flowers. I associate mulberries with summertime: memories of summer nights spent chasing fireflies, playing kickball on our dead-end street, riding bikes, playing in the sprinkler and, of course — picking mulberries. What we didn't eat, my sister and I and our neighborhood friends would crush with a brick, add a little water and paint monochromatic pictures using mulberry paint. Life was good.

Mulberry trees can be found throughout the US, typically in warmer climates. Different species grow around the world. Their origins can be traced to eastern Asia, Africa and even North America.

These days I am a little savvier on just how special mulberries are. Historically, mulberries were made into jams, jellies, wines and pies and used as folk medicine to treat coughs, colds and respiratory infections. They are highly nutritious and packed with calcium, phosphorus, magnesium and potassium. Mulberry leaves can be cooked or dried to make tea and help the body to process sugars. They are used in Chinese herbal medicine as a liver tonic.

Mulberries tend to be dark purple and even black when ripe; other mulberries are actually white when ripe. To prevent bruising, harvest by pinching and twisting the stem with one hand while holding the branch with the other. They are highly perishable, so use them right away or freeze them for later use.

I like to make honey mulberry jam, popsicles, smoothies, popovers and chocolate-covered mulberries. One of my very favorite recipes is a decadent raw mulberry cheesecake with a fig and almond crust and cashew crème as the cheesecake filling — an embodiment of summer. The richness of the cashew crème is cut perfectly with the lemon and mulberry pairings. The figs bring out a sweet earthy flavor, and the almonds provide the perfect crunch for the crust. The sweet drizzle on top rounds out the dish, making it both a decadent and refreshing summertime dessert. (See page 161 for the recipe.)

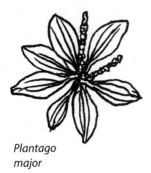

Plantago major

Plantain has been used throughout history as a panacea, meaning a medicine that is used to treat everything. It has antibacterial, astringent and anti-in-flammatory properties. Young leaves can be eaten raw and are loaded with vitamin C and calcium. Plantain is one of the main ingredients in first-aid salve. To treat insect stings quickly, simply pluck a leaf of plantain, tear it apart and use a little saliva to make an instant paste. Hold it on the sting for at least a minute.

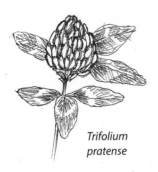

Trifolium pratense

Red clover is a wonderful weed that grows wild in pastures and fields worldwide. Native to western Asia, Europe and Africa, it is a wonderful women's health herb as it is a source of phytoestrogens, plant-based estrogens. It can aid in menstrual cramps, PMS, hot flashes and other symptoms of menopause. Red clover can also be helpful in treating the common cold and flu, as it helps loosen phlegm, and is good for the heart, keeping arteries flexible. It is rich in vitamins and minerals including calcium, potassium, magnesium and vitamin C.

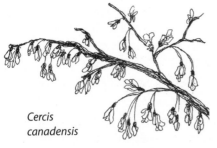

Cercis canadensis

Redbud trees, native to the Eastern US, are one of the first trees to bloom in the early spring, late March to early

May. The purple redbud flowers, rich in vitamin C, can be collected and eaten raw. I like to add them to a foraged salad of dandelion greens, young plantain, young sassafras leaves and wild onion. Dry them to make a lovely floral tea or add to water and freeze into pretty ice cubes.

Stinging nettles, native to North America, Asia, Europe and Africa, grow wild in woodlands, prairies and savannahs. It can be hard to distinguish between wood nettles and false nettles. In fact, for years I had been confusing stinging nettles with wood nettles (which are also highly medicinal) until an herbalist friend described their differences. Stinging nettle leaves have a very distinct pattern of three major veins running lengthwise down the center. The leaf pattern is opposite and the leaves are lanceolate. Wood nettles have more ovular leaves with a pinnate

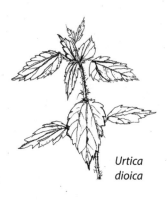

Urtica dioica

venation. Also, their bottom leaves are alternate, and their top leaves are opposite. The stinging hairs that run the entire length of the stem cause an immediate burning and itching reaction in the skin. Some herbalists intentionally run their hands and arms into a stinging nettle patch as a successful method of treating arthritis.

Nettles are one of the most amazing medicinal herbs. They are used to treat cold and flu, digestive upsets and skin disorders and are a good tonic for the urinary tract, kidneys, heart and lungs. Stinging nettles are also revered as a wild edible, eaten by Native Americans for their high nutrient content and are rich in iron, potassium, calcium and vitamin C. The young leaves can be eaten fresh, but they must be folded to reduce the risk of stinging while chewing or swallowing. The leaves may be soaked in water to remove the stingers. Substitute them for spinach in any dish. One of the most creative dishes I have ever enjoyed was stinging nettle gnocchi, from our friends at Kitchen Kulture.

Wild onions can be found in the spring and summer throughout the US. They look like grass but are hollow and tubular, found in clusters and have a very potent onion flavor. Use them just as you would chives, scallions or onions. Cut with scissors and serve raw in salad,

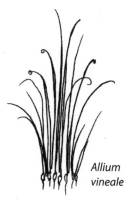

Allium vineale

cooked with meals or added to flavor sauces and soups. Wild onion soup is delicious served with wild onion biscuits.

Onions have been used historically to treat respiratory infections. They contain high anticancer sulfur compounds and help regulate healthy cholesterol levels.

Spring Tonic Tea Blend

¼ cup burdock root (fresh or dried)
¼ cup dandelion leaves (fresh)
⅛ cup dandelion root (fresh or dried)
⅛ cup echinacea root (fresh or dried)
⅛ cup ginger root (fresh or dried)
¼ cup nettle leaf
⅛ cup red clover blossoms
2 gallons water

Boil water and pour over herbs. Let steep for 5 minutes. Let cool. Strain herbs. Store in the refrigerator up to 4 days. Drink a cup in the morning, one in the afternoon and another in the evening.

Foraging and Cultivating Mushrooms

Foraging Mushrooms

Wild mushroom hunting is a highly rewarding outdoor activity. It is crucial to buy a regional or state guide in order to properly identify and distinguish edible mushrooms from poisonous look alikes. Get involved with your local mycology association or chapter.

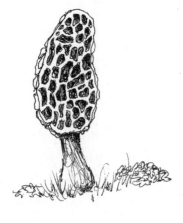

Our favorite mushrooms are the mighty morels that are prolific in the Mississippi River valley. They are a prized possession indeed! We enjoy finding just enough to eat and share. They have a unique rich flavor and simply wonderful texture and are excellent stuffed with goat cheese and wild onions.

Chicken of the woods mushrooms are thick, hard and spongy. They are bright orange and are often found growing on fallen decomposing trees. We love to make fried chicken of the woods with herb cashew ranch dipping sauce.

Among our favorite foraged mushrooms are oyster mushrooms, hen of the woods, chanterelles and dryad's saddle. We tend to stick to just a few different types per year, to be sure that we can properly identify them and have time to study their environment. Resources available for edible mushrooms and mushroom identification throughout the US include state extension offices, departments of natural resources and mycology clubs.

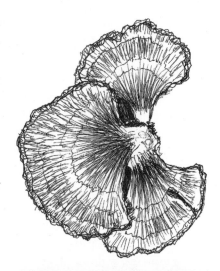

Mushroom Inoculation

Mushroom inoculation can be done easily at home. Several DIY tutorial videos are available online. We have successfully inoculated logs with shitakes, chicken of the woods, oyster mushrooms and reishi mushrooms. Logs already inoculated with spores can be purchased and have good results, but with shorter periods of harvest time. Mushrooms can also be inoculated in straw and grown inside laundry baskets. This is one of the most exciting ways I have seen mushrooms grow. To order supplies, visit fieldforest. net or fungi.com.

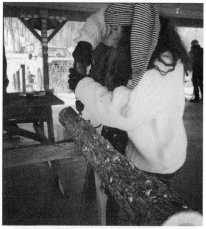

My husband and I attended a workshop put on by our friends at Goods from the Woods. We helped inoculate dozens of logs with mushroom spores, then coated them with beeswax and let them cure outside in the shade. We add new mushroom logs to our backyard each year.

We also participated in a workshop, presented by the McCully Heritage Project and led by Michelle Berg Vogel, based on the tutorials from Field & Forest

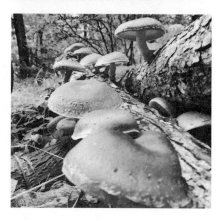

Products, an excellent resource for mushroom spores. We inoculated mushrooms using the following three methods.

Inoculating a Mushroom Log with Plugs (Early to Late Spring)

You will need several logs, ideally red or white oak, but sugar maple and sweetgum would also work, preferably from live healthy trees. We tend to go for live trees that have fallen from a storm or in an area of the forest that needs to be thinned in order to promote the growth of healthy native trees. The logs should be between 4 and 8 inches in diameter and nearly 3½ feet long.

You also need a cordless drill and a drill bit roughly the same size as your plug spawn or thimble spawn. Spawns come in different sizes. Mark your bit at one inch with a piece of tape to drill holes that deep. Drill holes into logs about 6 inches apart in 2 or 3 rows. Inoculate them with shitake plugs with a foam seal or dowel plugs and brush melted beeswax over them. Be sure to label your logs with the date, type of spawn and other pertinent information. Store them in a north-facing shady area of your yard. The ideal temperature range is 60° to 85°F. Logs should be stored horizontally and watered regularly to prevent them from drying out. Place them a couple of inches off the ground to permit air flow and to prevent them from being immersed in standing water.

It could be up to one year before the logs set fruit (produce mushrooms). Check them regularly and make a note of when they fruit. Mark your calendar for the following year so you will know when to expect them. The logs will fruit from anywhere between 2 and 8 years.

Growing Oyster Mushrooms on a Stump Using the Totem Method

(Adapted from tutorial by Field & Forest Products)

You will need:

> 6 logs between 6 and 12 inches in diameter and 12 to 16 inches long
> 6 2-inch slices of the same stump (carefully cut with a chainsaw)
> 6 black plastic bags without fungicide
> Sawdust inoculated with mushrooms (sawdust spawn):
> 2½ pounds of sawdust spawn should inoculate roughly 6 logs
> 12 to 24 sheets of black and white newspaper
> 6 large heavy-duty rubber bands

Open the plastic bag and spread about 1 cup of sawdust spawn at the bottom of the bag until it is roughly an 8-inch circle. Place the large stump on top of the spawn in the bag. Spread about 2 cups of sawdust spawn evenly onto the top of the log (it should be about ¼-inch thick). Add the 2-inch slice of log. Spread 2 cups of sawdust spawn evenly on top of this layer. Cover with 2 or 3 sheets of newspaper and fasten with a rubber band.

There should be 3 total layers of sawdust inoculated with oyster spores between the components: in the bag underneath the stump, between the stump and the stump slice and on the top of the stump slice.

Tie up the bag and place in a shady area of your basement for roughly 4 months. The ideal temperature for inoculation is between 60° and 80°F. Move it outside into a shady location and remove from the bag. The log should fruit in late summer to early fall. Check logs regularly. They will continue to produce for 2 more years. Repeat the steps every 2 years to ensure a yearly mushroom harvest.

Tee Pee Oyster Kit

Another simple way to grow oyster mushrooms (especially with kids) is using toilet paper rolls and the Tee Pee Oyster Kit from Field & Forest. Their 7-roll kit includes instructions as well as a 2-pound bag of oyster mushroom grain spawn, 7 filter bags and 7 rubber bands.

Fill a large pot halfway with water and bring to a boil. Remove from heat. Clean work surface. Using a pair of tongs, dip toilet paper rolls one at a time into the boiled water until fully saturated. Place them on a rack to drain and cool. When cooled, transfer one to each filter bag.

Shake the bag of spawn until the grains have separated. Cut a small opening in the corner of the spawn bag and carefully fill each of the inside tubes of the toilet paper rolls with the grain. Close each bag with a rubber band above the filter patch. Place the bags in a dark area where the temperature is between 65° and 75°F. Within 3 weeks, a white coating, the mycelium, should appear. Let it grow for 1 to 3 more weeks. Four to 6 weeks after inoculation, place in the refrigerator for 48 hours. Then remove and place in a sunny area at room temperature. Remove rubber bands and open the bags. Within 1 to 2 weeks, you should see the first mushrooms. Spray with water while they are developing. When they are about 2 inchs wide, twist the base to harvest. Rinse well.

After you harvest, close the bag again, place in a dark area and repeat the process about 2 or 3 more times. Compost toilet paper roll when no more mushrooms appear (after your third harvest).

Ozark Forest Mushrooms, owned by Dan and Nicola MacPherson, is a 3,500-acre family-owned farm in the Missouri Ozarks in an area that has been designated as one of the "Last Great Places" by the Nature Conservancy. It's an amazing example of how a business can be formed by growing and selling quality fresh mushrooms to restaurants, stores and individuals at farmers' markets. They practice healthy forest ecology while growing and harvesting a renewable supply of mushroom bed logs. They use draft horses to naturally thin their forests under the Missouri Department of Conservation guidelines. This farm produces delicious mushrooms as well as value-added products. They have been advocates of the local foods movement for decades and continue to do their part in helping to create localized food systems.

In 2008, mycologist and inventor Paul Stamets gave one of the most moving and captivating TED Talks of all time. This talk has inspired individuals and communities around the globe to think about and put into action mycoremediation. This talk will be marked in history as the foundation for groundbreaking scientific research. Paul Stamets is one of my greatest heroes! His work is profound, and the inspiration he provides spans the globe.

The following is a transcript directly from his TED Talk.

> I want to present to you a suite of six mycological solutions, using fungi, and these solutions are based on mycelium. The mycelium infuses all landscapes, it holds soils together, it's extremely tenacious. This holds up to 30,000 times its mass. They're the grand molecular disassemblers of nature — the soil magicians. They generate the humus soils across the landmasses of Earth. We have now discovered that there is a multi-directional transfer of nutrients between plants, mitigated by the mycelium — so the mycelium is the mother that is giving nutrients from alder and birch trees to hemlocks, cedars and Douglas firs. Mushrooms are very fast in their growth. Mushrooms produce strong antibiotics. In fact, we're more closely related to fungi than we are to any other kingdom. A group of 20 eukaryotic microbiologists published a paper two years ago erecting opisthokonta — a super-kingdom that joins animalia and fungi together. We share in common the same pathogens. Fungi don't like to rot from bacteria, and so our best antibiotics come from fungi. But here is a mushroom that's past its prime. After they sporulate, they do rot. But I propose to you that the sequence of

microbes that occur on rotting mushrooms are essential for the health of the forest. They give rise to the trees, they create the debris fields that feed the mycelium. In a single cubic inch of soil, there can be more than eight miles of these cells. My foot is covering approximately 300 miles of mycelium. I've been a scanning electron microscopist for many years, I have thousands of electron micrographs, and when I'm staring at the mycelium, I realize that they are microfiltration membranes. We exhale carbon dioxide, so does mycelium. It inhales oxygen, just like we do. But these are essentially externalized stomachs and lungs. And I present to you a concept that these are extended neurological membranes. And in these cavities, these micro-cavities form, and as they fuse soils, they absorb water. These are little wells. And inside these wells, then microbial communities begin to form. And so the spongy soil not only resists erosion, but sets up a microbial universe that gives rise to a plurality of other organisms. I first proposed, in the early 1990s, that mycelium is Earth's natural Internet. When you look at the mycelium, they're highly branched. And if there's one branch that is broken, then very quickly, because of the nodes of crossing — Internet engineers maybe call them hot points — there are alternative pathways for channeling nutrients and information. The mycelium is sentient. It knows that you are there. When you walk across landscapes, it leaps up in the aftermath of your footsteps trying to grab debris. So, I believe the invention of the computer Internet is an inevitable consequence of a previously proven, biologically successful model. The Earth invented the computer Internet for its own benefit, and we now, being the top organism on this planet, are trying to allocate resources in order to protect the biosphere. Going way out, dark matter conforms to the same mycelial archetype. I believe matter begets life; life becomes single cells; single cells become strings; strings become chains; chains network. And this is the paradigm that we see throughout the universe. Most of you may not know that fungi were the first organisms to come to land. They came to land 1.3 billion years ago, and plants followed several hundred million years later. How is that possible? It's possible because the mycelium produces oxalic acids, and many other acids and enzymes, pockmarking rock and grabbing calcium and other minerals and forming calcium oxalates. Makes the rocks crumble, and the first step in the generation of soil. Oxalic acid is two carbon dioxide molecules joined together. So, fungi and mycelium sequester carbon dioxide in the form of calcium oxalates. And all sorts of other oxalates are also sequestering carbon dioxide through the minerals that are being formed and taken out of the rock matrix. This was first discovered in 1859. A photograph was taken 1950s in Saudi Arabia. 420 million years ago, an organism existed — Prototaxites. Prototaxites, laying down, was about three feet tall. The tallest plants on Earth at that time were less than two feet. Dr. Boyce, at the University of Chicago, published an article in the *Journal of Geology* determining that Prototaxites was a giant fungus, a giant mushroom. Across the landscapes of Earth were dotted these giant mushrooms. All across most land masses. And these existed for tens of millions of years. Now, we've had several extinction events, and as we march forward — 65 million years ago — most of you know about it — we had an asteroid impact. The Earth was struck by an asteroid, a huge amount of debris was jettisoned into the atmosphere. Sunlight was cut off, and fungi inherited the Earth. Those organisms that paired with fungi were rewarded, because fungi do not need light. More recently, at Einstein University, they just determined that fungi use radiation as a source of energy, much like plants use light. So, the prospect of fungi existing on other planets elsewhere, I think, is a forgone conclusion, at least in my own mind. The largest organism in the world is in Eastern Oregon. I couldn't miss it. It was 2,200 acres in size: 2,200 acres in size, 2,000 years old. The largest organism on the planet is a mycelial mat, one cell wall thick. How is it that this organism can be so large, and yet be one cell wall thick, whereas we have five or six skin layers that protect us? The mycelium, in the right conditions, produces a mushroom — it bursts through with such ferocity that it can break asphalt. We were involved with several experiments. I'm going to show you six, if I can, solutions for helping to save the world. Battelle Laboratories and I joined up in Bellingham, Washington. There were four piles saturated with diesel and other petroleum waste: one was a control pile;

one pile was treated with enzymes; one pile was treated with bacteria; and our pile we inoculated with mushroom mycelium. The mycelium absorbs the oil. The mycelium is producing enzymes — peroxidases — that break carbon-hydrogen bonds. These are the same bonds that hold hydrocarbons together. So, the mycelium becomes saturated with the oil, and then, when we returned six weeks later, all the tarps were removed, all the other piles were dead, dark and stinky. We came back to our pile, it was covered with hundreds of pounds of oyster mushrooms, and the color changed to a light form. The enzymes remanufactured the hydrocarbons into carbohydrates — fungal sugars. Some of these mushrooms are very happy mushrooms. They're very large. They're showing how much nutrition that they could've obtained. But something else happened, which was an epiphany in my life. They sporulated, the spores attract insects, the insects laid eggs, eggs became larvae. Birds then came, bringing in seeds, and our pile became an oasis of life. Whereas the other three piles were dead, dark and stinky, and the PAH's — the aromatic hydrocarbons — went from 10,000 parts per million to less than 200 in eight weeks. The last image we don't have. The entire pile was a green berm of life. These are gateway species, vanguard species that open the door for other biological communities. So I invented burlap sacks, bunker spawn — and putting the mycelium — using storm blown debris, you can take these burlap sacks and put them downstream from a farm that's producing E. coli, or other wastes, or a factory with chemical toxins, and it leads to habitat restoration. So, we set up a site in Mason County, Washington, and we've seen a dramatic decrease in the amount of coliforms. And I'll show you a graph here. This is a logarithmic scale, 10 to the eighth power. There's more than a 100 million colonies per gram, and 10 to the third power is around 1,000. In 48 hours to 72 hours, these three mushroom species reduced the amount of coliform bacteria 10,000 times. Think of the implications. This is a space-conservative method that uses storm debris — and we can guarantee that we will have storms every year.

So, this one mushroom, in particular, has drawn our interest over time. Agarikon is a mushroom exclusive to the old-growth forest that Dioscorides first described in 65 AD as a treatment against consumption. This mushroom grows in Washington State, Oregon, northern California, British Columbia, now thought to be extinct in Europe. May not seem that large — let's get closer. This is extremely rare fungus. Our team — and we have a team of experts that go out — we went out 20 times in the old-growth forest last year. We found one sample to be able to get into culture. Preserving the genome of these fungi in the old-growth forest I think is absolutely critical for human health. I've been involved with the US Defense Department BioShield program. We submitted over 300 samples of mushrooms that were boiled in hot water, and mycelium harvesting these extracellular metabolites. And a few years ago, we received these results. We have three different strains of Agarikon mushrooms that were highly active against poxviruses. Dr. Earl Kern, who's a smallpox expert of the US Defense Department, states that any compounds that have a selectivity index of two or more are active. 10 or greater are considered to be very active. Our mushroom strains were in the highly active range.

So, encouraged by this, naturally we went to flu viruses. And so, for the first time, I am showing this. We have three different strains of Agarikon mushrooms highly active against flu viruses. Here's the selectivity index numbers — against pox, you saw 10s and 20s — now against flu viruses, compared to the ribavirin controls, we have an extraordinarily high activity. And we're using a natural extract within the same dosage window as a pure pharmaceutical. We tried it against flu A viruses — H1N1, H3N2 — as well as flu B viruses. So then we tried a blend, and in a blend combination we tried it against H5N1, and we got greater than 1,000 selectivity index. I then think that we can make the argument that we should save the old-growth forest as a matter of national defense.

I became interested in entomopathogenic fungi — fungi that kill insects. Our house was being destroyed by carpenter ants. So, I went to the EPA homepage, and they were recommending studies with metarhizium species of a group of fungi that kill carpenter ants, as well as termites. I did something that nobody else had done. I actually chased the mycelium, when it stopped producing spores. These are spores — this is in their spores. I was able to morph the culture into a non-sporulating form. And so the industry has spent over 100 million dollars specifically on bait stations to prevent termites from eating your house. But the insects aren't stupid, and they would avoid the spores when they came close, and so I morphed the cultures into a non-sporulating form. And I got my daughter's Barbie doll dish, I put it right where a bunch of carpenter ants were making debris fields, every day, in my house, and the ants were attracted to the mycelium, because there's no spores. They gave it to the queen. One week later, I had no sawdust piles whatsoever.

And then — a delicate dance between dinner and death — the mycelium is consumed by the ants, they become mummified, and, boing, a mushroom pops out of their head. Now after sporulation, the spores repel. So, the house is no longer suitable for invasion. So, you have a near-permanent solution for reinvasion of termites. And so my house came down, I received my first patent against carpenter ants, termites and fire ants. Then we tried extracts, and lo and behold, we can steer insects to different directions. This has huge implications. I then received my second patent — and this is a big one. It's been called an Alexander Graham Bell patent. It covers over 200,000 species. This is the most disruptive technology — I've been told by executives of the pesticide industry — that they have ever witnessed. This could totally revamp the pesticide industries throughout the world. You could fly 100 PhD students under the umbrella of this concept, because my supposition is that entomopathogenic fungi, prior to sporulation, attract the very insects that are otherwise repelled by those spores.

And so I came up with a Life Box, because I needed a delivery system. The Life Box: you add soil, you add water, you have mycorrhizal and endophytic fungi as well as spores, like of the Agarikon mushroom. The seeds then are mothered by this mycelium. And then you put tree seeds in here, and then you end up growing — potentially — an old-growth forest from a cardboard box. I want to reinvent the delivery system, and the use of cardboard around the world, so they become ecological footprints. You could take a cardboard box delivering shoes, you could add water — I developed this for the refugee community — corns, beans and squash and onions. I took several containers and I ended up growing a seed garden. Then you harvest the seeds — and thank you and then you're harvesting the seed garden. Then you can harvest the kernels, and then you just need a few kernels. I add mycelium to it, and then I inoculate the corncobs. Now, three corncobs, no other grain — lots of mushrooms begin to form. Too many withdrawals from the carbon bank, and so this population will be shut down. But watch what happens here. The mushrooms then are harvested, but very importantly, the mycelium has converted the cellulose into fungal sugars. And so I thought, how could we address the energy crisis in this country?

And we came up with Econol. Generating ethanol from cellulose using mycelium as an intermediary — and you gain all the benefits that I've described to you already. But to go from cellulose to ethanol is ecologically unintelligent, and I think that we need to be econologically intelligent about the generation of fuels. So, we build the carbon banks on the planet, renew the soils. These are a species that we need to join with. I think engaging mycelium can help save the world.

— Paul Stamets
TED Talk 2008 "Six Ways Mushrooms Can Save the World"

Paul Stamets is an environmental crusader and a true steward of the Earth. His work is extremely important to solution-based practices facing the major environmental concerns of our time. His work could change the future of the planet. He is also well-versed in how mushrooms can be used in bioremediation and environmental cleanup; filtration of water and wastewater; reforestation; sustainable agriculture; as medicine and emergency food; as natural pesticides; and in the production of biofuels. Visit his website fungi.com to learn more.

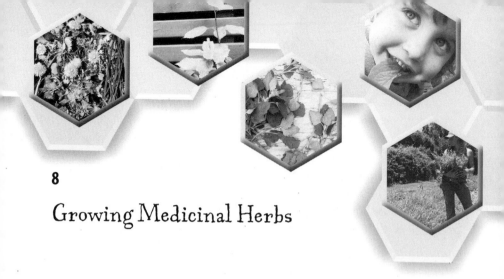

8

Growing Medicinal Herbs

M Y FIRST INTRODUCTION TO MEDICINAL HERBS was the summer my American literature and journalism instructor, Byron Clemens, invited me to accompany him and his wife, Beatrice, on a family trip to Big Mountain, Arizona, in the Former Joint Use Area of the Hopi and Navajo Indian Reservation. Big Mountain is held sacred by several southwestern indigenous nations. It is considered the spiritual altar between the four sacred mountains. They had been advocating for social justice and environmental policies on the reservation for years. They dedicated countless hours of volunteer time bringing supplies to the reservation, organizing groups to lend support and to protest Peabody Coal. I was honored when they asked me to accompany them as their children's nanny during the summer of 1998. While there, the local medicine man asked me to assist with him in the med-

ical tent at the Sundance (put on by the Lakota people for the Navajo and Hopi). I considered it a great privilege and honor to assist in making foot baths for the dancers (using local creosote brush) and in preparing herbal medicine, collecting wild plants and infusing them in oils and alcohols to make muscle rubs and tinctures. Witnessing the Sundance and being asked to lend a hand in the medical tent were experiences that have sculpted and enriched my life in many ways. The smell of the white sage and cedar burning struck me with a wave

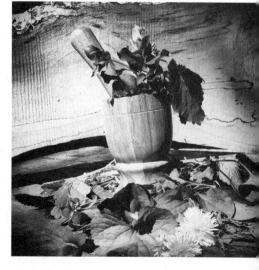

of emotion, awakening my every sense. The sound of sacred songs and drum-
ming echoed amongst the fragrant junipers and pines. The beautiful, insistent
beating of the drum seemed to capture Mother Earth's very own heartbeat.
The dancers exuded an energy beyond this dimension. Their strength and
resilience humbled me and prompted deep self-reflection. I felt a sense of
visceral connectedness to the land. To witness the prayer, ritual, wisdom,
sacrifice and stoic beauty was such an honor. A sacred tree was placed in the
middle of the Sundance circle where the dancers, long strands attaching them
to the tree, made flesh offerings to the creator. Barefoot and in rhythm with
the elements, they fasted and prayed and remained strong. From the branches of the trees hung thousands of tiny satchels, their colors representing the
four sacred directions. They contained offerings of tobacco and sage and were
infused by members of the tribe with prayers and pleas. These hung from
the tree and blew in the wind. I learned of the Navajo Beauty Way, which
was also respected and revered by the Hopi tribe. I touched the ancient and
energetically charged Hopi Prophecy Rock. I was witness to the magnificent
desert landscape painted with picturesque colors of the Southwest: terra cotta
red sandstone, blue-gray hues of sagebrush, salt brush, cacti, pinon trees contrasted with the black veins of coal running through the plateaus, heavenly
blue skies and the tan and white tones of the barren earth.

Big Mountain, where the mountain lions, coyotes and prairie rattlesnakes
take the reins of their predatory roles. Big Mountain, where the sky is so vast
with brushstrokes of vivid blue that you can see the geology of the land for
miles and miles; where you can see the red-tailed hawks, golden eagles, prairie falcons, crows and American kestrels soaring the skies, hunting jackrabbits

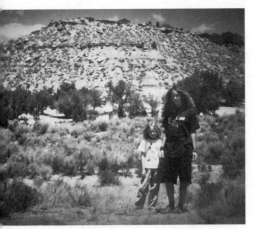

and a wide array of small animals and
vertebrates scattered throughout the
landscape; where if you listen closely
you can hear sounds of coyotes and
owls play a haunting soundtrack to the
hushed stories of things that should
not be named that roam the inverted
valley at night. One finds comfort in
the blanket of stars covering the night
sky, flickering for eons ... their bright-
ness brilliant against the illusion of the
pitch black backdrop of space. I had
never seen the stars so bright and the

sky so black. It left me to ponder Olbers' paradox, the mystery of why the sky is dark at night when there are an infinite number of stars that should theoretically light it up. The trip to Big Mountain made a lasting impression on me. Learning about plant medicine laid the framework for the beginning of my journey with medicinal herbs.

A trip to Costa Rica as a high-school senior changed my life even further and deepened my connection to nature in a profound way, as I became familiar with permaculture for the very first time at Punta Mona Center for Sustainability. Bathing in the cool waters of the La Fortuna waterfall by day and soaking in the warm hot springs at the base of the glowing Arenal Volcano by night truly left me speechless. Learning of some of the most medicinal plants in the rainforest, and possibly the world, such as noni, star fruit, turmeric and ginger, expanded my understanding of the important role food plays in our health.

In 2000, I received news that my father was diagnosed with lung cancer and was told he had six months to live. This event led me to put into practice my interest in alternative medicine.

As believers in natural healthcare, my mother and I took part in convincing him to adopt alternative medicine and to avoid chemotherapy and radiation for as long as possible. I got a job at a local health food store in order to receive the discount on organic foods, herbs and supplements. I worked in the juice bar and would bring him wheatgrass shots and fresh pressed vegetable juices after each shift. I remember reading articles on juicing and wheatgrass in a *Mother Earth News* magazine and learning their benefits to the systems of the body. My mother and I started cooking healthier meals. We limited our intake of salt, sugar, saturated fats and processed foods. We followed advice from several books on nutrition and herbal remedies. My father's energy level significantly increased with each natural approach we took. He started seeing an acupuncturist, Dr. Sachs. He began taking a plethora of Chinese herbal remedies such as reishi mushrooms. He showed tremendous results from these treatments, which kept him alive five years longer than the doctors had expected.

My father's story is one of many that keep the healing power of plants alive by inspiring new herbalists and alternative medicine practitioners, as well as reaffirming the goals of those who have trusted in plants to heal people for many moons. These medicinal plants and their true healing powers have been revered since the dawn of humanity, but unfortunately have somehow become lost knowledge in our modern world. Western society tends to rely exclusively on the advances of Western medicine and technological approaches to treatment.

My father's story and the encouragement of my friend Colleen inspired me to begin my studies as an herbalist through the American College of Health Science (formerly Australasian College of Herbal Studies).

Healing plants are all around us. In fact, there are over 400,000 known species, and more are discovered and documented every day. Learning to identify these sacred plants and their individual capacities for healing is an art form and a beautiful process. Identifying a single plant in a forest setting is like recognizing and being able to spot a friend in a large crowd of people. It makes sense to me that individuals you can recognize after a chance second meeting are more than likely individuals that you connected with on the first meeting. This can be applied energetically to the plant world. Plants that you recognize are oftentimes plants that can be useful to you in some fashion or another. However, it is a lifelong journey, given how many species there are; the most important ones to start with are the highly medicinal plants as well as the highly poisonous plants within your specific region. During my herb workshops, I encourage individuals to start learning to identify the plants growing in their own backyard and neighborhood.

Throughout my herbal path, I kept hearing the name Rosemary Gladstar. First, what a wonderful name! I soon realized Rosemary Gladstar is a world-renowned herbalist and author. After we met in person at the Mother Earth News Fair, she has become my hero — a wonder woman, a wizard of the woods, a Van Gogh in her garden and an absolute gem of a human being. Rosemary is one of those individuals who is so warm and welcoming that she makes you feel like family. Her smile lights up a room, and just being in viewing distance of her is uplifting. I am so glad that she is on the forefront of herbalism today because she is a perfect and radiant example of how both plants and humans should hold each other in genuine reverence. She is a living, breathing example of the type of personality that could arise as the result of a paradigm shift. She offers herbal education. Check her out at sagemountain.com.

Numen: The Nature of Plants, a Film Review

In my experience with plants as both a grower and an herbalist, I have seen firsthand the healing power of plants time and time again, and it never ceases to amaze me. The vigor and vibrancy of plants is magical. They are one of the greatest life forces on Earth and inherently hold the key to our well-being. Plants nourish our bodies inside and out.

Numen

Numen: The Nature of Plants, a film by Brook Hollow Productions, created by Ann Armbrecht and Terrence Youk in association with United Plant Savers, is a cornucopia of intuitive wisdom, scientific knowledge, exuberant passion and reverence for plants around the world. The film is dedicated to and in memory of the late Bill Mitchell, co-founder of Bastyr University. The film opens with plant close-ups and stunning time-lapse photography of plants throughout their growing cycles, their intrinsic eye-catching patterns and their symbiotic relationships with pollinators.

"Numen" is defined as the spirit believed by animists to inhabit natural objects. The film describes how we sense this force the most abundantly through plants. I immediately visualized the life cycle of the sunflower. When you close your eyes and imagine one sunflower seed in the palm of your hand, you notice the shape, the size, the texture, the color, the pattern and striations. Imagine placing it in soil and seeing the sprout cracking out of its shell. The roots push their way down into the rich dark earth at the same time the sprout forms a stem and cotyledons appear like magic. The stem stretches for the sun and begins to grow wider and taller. Leaves form and the stout square stem burrows strong roots into the earth. Soft rains fall. The stem grows and grows and new leaves form. The bud forms. The leaves once protecting the fragile bud begin to fold back, exposing the inward-facing petals to the sunlight. The sunflower's tight bud slowly begins to blossom, a process which can occur within just a few hours. The bloom opens wide, fully embracing the life force energy of the sun, even turning with it. The sunflower proudly displays its inherent sacred geometry, the Fibonacci spiral. As it is meant to, it fulfills the very essence of its being, welcoming pollinators to drink its sweet nectar in the mutually beneficial relationship that is pollination. The sunflower, whose petals capture the very essence of the sun itself, whose sight is stunning against the backdrop of a clear blue sky, whose company is pleasant as it dances in the gentle breeze throughout changing seasons. As it fulfills the very nature of its purposeful life cycle, seeds form and become food for humans, small animals and birds alike.

Numen describes the intelligent and intuitive characteristics each plant intrinsically holds. Indeed the animated life force is recognizable in plants, if we take the time to notice their beauty and magic. Their shapes, sizes, colors, textures, heights determine their vastly unique characteristics. Just as we recognize unique personality and character traits in our loved ones, like a unique laugh, the color of their hair, their vibrant eyes and their smile, so too can we learn to notice and celebrate the individual characteristics of every plant. Identifying and getting to know plants can be seen in the same light. Recognizing a plant just as you would a friend is an excellent way to delve into the vast art of plant medicine, foraging, gardening and plant science.

When considering the most fundamental building block of life on Earth, Kenny Ausubel, founder of Bioneers, eloquently makes a critical point that "the history of humanity is the history of our relationship to plants." Dr. Tieraona Low Dog points out the simple yet precise fact that "all people historically and today have relied on plants for their food, medicine and clothing." Dr. Rocio Alarcon, an ethnobotanist, is fascinated by the notion that "humans have been living approximately only 5 million years; agriculture has been around for only 10,000 years; plants have been around for 400 million years. You can imagine the evolution of these plants to have these incredible rich properties."

Rosemary Gladstar explains how "herbalism is the oldest system of healing used on the planet; plants are our teachers and we have evolved in relation to them; everything at the base of the food chain comes from plants. Plants were here long before humans and we have evolved in relationship to them." Dr. Hellen Oketch, chief scientist at Herb Pharm, points out that "plants are the only organism that are able to transmit the energy from the source (the sun) into a form that can be used by humans" and also states that "some of the biochemistry found in plants is similar to some of the biochemistry found in humans." Herbalist and healer Raylene Ha'aleelea Kawaiae'a believes that "plants are our ancestors, our elders" and that "we should treat our elders well and respect them dearly because they have wisdom to share with us." Bill Mitchell, ND and co-founder of Bastyr University, concludes that "our DNA contains so much material from the plant world. A lot of the DNA, the memory, comes from the very origins of life. When life was evolving, most of the green material found in the ocean consisted of omega-3 oils, the chloroplasts, omega-3 oils that seem to be the fundamental oil of the universe. The body still needs omega-3 oils, as they are the substrate to many chemical reactions. So we are connected to the beginning of life itself." Matthew Wood, clinical herbalist, states that "in the 19th century, herbalism was really part of the marrow of American society and was deeply entrenched," and explained that 90% of the population knew how to treat themselves with herbs.

The film describes how, in the late 1890s and the early 1900s in North America, you could walk into any drugstore and buy hundreds of herbal products, especially liquid herbal extracts. Ausubel explains that "many major natural medicine traditions going back, are all founded in these basic principles that nature is the source of healing." He goes on to explain a divergence, a conflict in medical philosophy between the natural medicine school and the conventional (allopathic) schools of medicine, that directly affected the future of healthcare in the US and around the world. What was once considered healthcare quickly became sickcare. Ed Smith explains how "natural medicine began to die out as folk medicine after World War II because people were enthralled with new science and technology and craved to be modern and how we are moving into a new era." Rosemary Gladstar notices that less than 100 years ago, people began to push pills instead of herbal medicine and vitamin supplements over fruits and vegetables. She explains that this modern medicine claimed to end disease and unfortunately influenced an entire generation to turn to Western medicine and completely dismiss thousands of years of herbal plant medicine.

The disconnection has developed out of the fact that we began to dissociate ourselves from where our food and medicine come from. This disassociation in turn fostered a mindset of disconnection between humans and nature. The sad effects of this massive disconnect is that we are now seeing a rise in chronic illnesses. We are moving farther and farther away from fresh air, clean water, healthy soil, safe food and ultimately our historic source for health and wellness, plants. Ausubel points out that "the huge toxicity directly related to drilling oil and all of the thousands of chemicals produced as derivatives are now poisoning the entire web of life, ourselves included. The whole idea of ecological medicine embodies that we are connected to the ecosystems around us and that we can only really be healthy when the land and the water around us are also healthy and if they are not, then it's going to show up in our physical well-being." Many of these ill effects are being researched and documented, author Mark Shapiro points out. The Centers for Disease Control surveyed a group of random Americans and found that the average American has 148 chemicals in their bloodstream. Dr. Martha Herbert, assistant professor of neurology at Harvard, states that these chemicals are "wreaking havoc at the molecular level and then that cascades up to the cellular and organism and ecosystem level." The film goes on to explain the detrimental effects humans have caused throughout the last century but also provides hope in offering practical solutions of which we are all capable of being a part. I have yet to see a film that sums all of these complex issues up as clearly as *Numen* does.

With all this knowledge about the current state of the environment, the world, we are faced with a personal decision. There is a severe dilemma ...

we must choose a healthier way for the future of the planet. We must make smarter choices about our food, choices about medicine. We must make decisions that will improve the quality of our lives, not decisions that will contribute to our demise.

The solutions the film outlines may be familiar: limit the use of plastics, shop local, buy local, adopt a diet that includes 70 percent vegetables, including dark leafy greens, a colorful array of fruits and vegetables and fresh herbs; avoid big-box stores; walk instead of drive; grow your own food and medicine; share your knowledge with your friends and neighbors; don't use toxic cleaners; reduce, reuse and recycle. The larger lesson is to make a conscious effort in our daily lives to understand the interconnectedness and symbiotic relationships occurring all around us — between people and the Earth, people and people, people and plants, people and animals, plants and animals, and all the connections in between. We then discover and implement ways of honoring these connections in our daily lives. It is up to every single one of us to make small changes and adapt for the greater good. Holding reverence for the very thing that brings nourishment to almost all life ... plants are the one thing that will truly open our eyes and hearts to healing ourselves and healing the Earth.

My Local Heroes

My dear friend Colleen Rena Smith shared my exuberance for plants and herbs and their healing abilities and seemed to be on a parallel path on the quest to learn about herbs. Her father had been growing medicinal herbs (bee balm and lemon balm) for many years. She was a catalyst in my life-long journey with herbs. On a summer road trip in 2000, she and I set out to see the western United States to visit our dream schools. I had my eye on Evergreen College in Olympia, Washington, and she wanted to visit the Australasian College of Herbal Studies. Colleen went on to apprentice with herbalists in Silver City, New Mexico, while I actually later pursued the Australasian College of Herbal Studies.

In my community, Cheryl Hoard owned and operated Cheryl's Herbs in St. Louis since 1991. She inspired many budding herbalists. Sadly, Cheryl passed away in 2015. She left a legacy by passing down herbal wisdom and the healing power of natural medicine to all those who knew her.

Another local hero of mine is Kristine Brown, creator and author of the *Herbal Roots* zine for kids. My children have enjoyed her great ideas, stories and crafts geared toward kids. They love integrating learning about the plants around them with educational projects. Kristine homeschools her children. They are already herbalists, learning from their mother all the beautiful ways that herbs can heal the land and its inhabitants. Her children have a respect for plants that is truly amazing to witness. It is a joy and an honor to know her and her family.

Growing Medicinal Herbs

> For all the types of pain that can lead to suffering there is a solution. Through opening our hearts with compassion to the pain that life brings, we can truly cure our pain and avoid our suffering. Then we can walk in the valley of love and experience the vast space within our heart.
>
> — Sebastian Pole

Some medicinal herbs are difficult to grow from seed. I recommend getting perennial divisions or cuttings from your local herbalist or herb-loving friend. To find a local herbalist, check with your local herb store, apothecary shop or health food store. A local herbalist is best found by word of mouth. Perennial divisions are simply a small portion of an established plant that is typically cut with a shovel (roots and all); the mother plant will still thrive. The perennial division can then be transplanted into a pot or directly into the ground. It will most likely take it a while to recover from transplant shock as it needs to get used to the new growing conditions. As long as it is buried deep enough and gets adequate sun and water, it should grow well. Some plant nurseries sell medicinal plant starts that can be directly transplanted into your medicinal herb garden.

Find here my top ten favorite medicinal herbs to grow and use. These can be found growing in the wild in this region or can be easily cultivated.

Borage (Annual that reseeds itself/Full sun/ Likes warmer weather)

Borage is a beautiful plant. Its young leaves and bluish-purple flowers are edible. It has been used medicinally since medieval times. Borage is known for its antidepressant and anti-inflammatory properties. Borage flowers are mostly used in salads and to decorate cupcakes, and they attract beneficial pollinators.

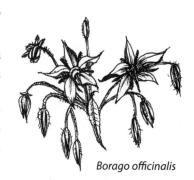

Borago officinalis

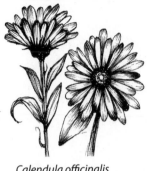

Calendula officinalis

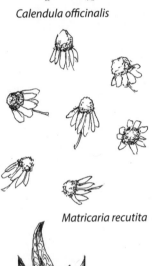

Matricaria recutita

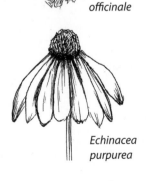

Symphytum officinale

Echinacea purpurea

Calendula (Annual that reseeds itself/ Full sun/Likes warmer weather).

Calendula is one of my favorite flowering herbs. Just like borage, calendula flowers are edible and make nice decorations to cakes and cupcakes. It accelerates healing and has been used to aid the lymphatic system. A healing first-aid salve can be made to help heal minor cuts and scrapes. Calendula is antifungal, anti-inflammatory, antimicrobial, and antispasmodic, and it is a known astringent, with diaphoretic properties.

Chamomile (Annual that reseeds itself/ Full sun & partial shade/Does well in moderate warm weather)

Chamomile flowers have one of the most magical aromas. It soothes the mind, body and spirit and is a mild sedative that helps aid in sleep. It can help alleviate headaches, skin rashes, digestive upsets and menstrual cramps. Chamomile is safe for children in small doses. It is anti-allergenic, antibacterial, anti-inflammatory, antifungal, antiseptic and antispasmodic.

Comfrey (Perennial/Full sun/Likes warmer weather)

Comfrey, with its serious healing powers, can be used topically for minor cuts, scrapes and wounds. It is the main ingredient in natural first-aid salves. It has many contraindications (inadvisable forms of treatment for a number of reasons) and should not be used internally. Comfrey tea makes a great natural garden fertilizer. Comfrey is alterative, astringent, demulcent, mucilaginous and nutritive.

Echinacea, Purple Coneflower (Perennial/Full sun/ Likes warmer weather)

Echinacea is an amazing medicinal herb. The whole plant can be used. As an herbalist, I have been making tinctures for years, and my favorite is an immune-strengthening tincture that includes echinacea. When made into a salve, echinacea can treat minor cuts, wounds, scrapes or burns.

We have planted several echinacea flowers in each of the places we have lived. It is among my favorite medicinal plants, helping to alleviate and reduce cold and flu symptoms and boost the immune system. Echinacea is anti-inflammatory, antiviral, antifungal, antibacterial and acts as a blood purifier.

Lavender (Tender perennial/Full sun/ Likes warmer weather)

Growing lavender feels like a sacred endeavor. It is such a healing and soothing flowering herb, and it has a calming aroma. Lavender can be used fresh or dried in teas. It has antibacterial, antifungal, antiseptic, anti-inflammatory and antidepressant properties.

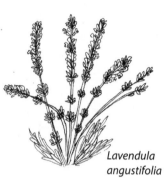

Lavendula angustifolia

St. John's Wort (Perennial/Full sun/ Likes warmer weather)

St. John's wort, a mood-enhancing and uplifting herb, is used to treat anxiety, sleep disorders and mild depression. It produces tiny yellow flowers that "bleed" red when crushed. St. John's wort is alterative, antifungal and antispasmodic and acts as an astringent, blood purifier, diuretic, nervine and sedative.

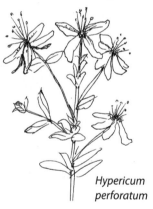

Hypericum perforatum

Tulsi (Holy basil) (Tender perennial/ Full sun/ Likes warmer weather)

Holy basil, an aromatic herb, has both culinary and medicinal value. Tulsi likely originated in India, where it is revered as an incarnation of the Hindu goddess, Tulsi. It plays an important role in Ayurvedic medicine. When made into a tea, holy basil can relieve cold and flu symptoms, reduce inflammation and reduce digestive upsets. Tulsi is antibacterial, antifungal, anti-inflammatory and antioxidant.

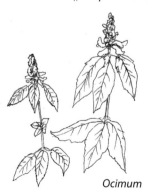

Ocimum

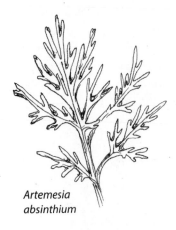

*Artemesia
absinthium*

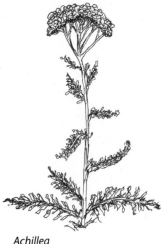

*Achillea
millefolium*

Wormwood (Perennial/Full sun/Likes warmer weather)

Wormwood, a spectacular silvery plant that grows extremely tall, is an anthelmintic herb that helps to expel parasites from the body. It is also used to treat a variety of digestive upsets including nausea and heartburn. Wormwood is anti-inflammatory, antipyretic, antiseptic and tonic.

Yarrow (Perennial/Full sun/Likes warmer weather)

Yarrow, a delicate-looking aromatic herb, can be used to stop bleeding. It has been used to treat cold and flu symptoms and is an effective blood cleanser. Yarrow is alterative, antiseptic, astringent, diaphoretic, homeostatic and a stimulant.

Read more about the uses for medicinal herbs in the **Create** section of this book.

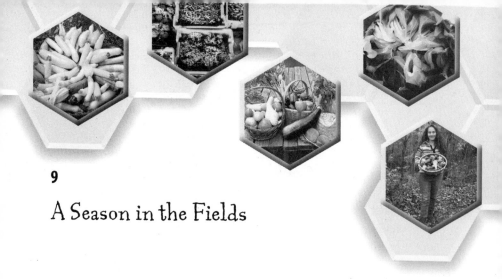

9

A Season in the Fields

Growing Together: Our Family's Anecdotes of Farming La Vista Farm

MY HUSBAND ERIC WAS HIRED as the head farmer at La Vista in February of 2010. And so the journey began: two ambitious plant enthusiasts, one sweet little nature boy and one beautiful farm sitting on the bluffs of the Mighty Mississippi. Eric had previous experience working on a farm. We jumped right into the sustainable farming process.

Community Gardens: A Love Affair with Plants Begins

Eric discovered his interest in vegetable gardening by joining a community garden in St. Louis, Missouri, while in college. I discovered my passion for planting when I did a seed starting science fair project in elementary school. Eric and I went from gardeners to farmers when he was hired to install several one acre community gardens as an AmeriCorps VISTA project in Salem, MO.

Sowing seeds in the high tunnel instantaneously became a part of who I am. It felt as though my purpose in life had been handed to me on a silver (or vibrant green) platter. Eric fell in love with the job immediately. When we weren't sowing thousands of seeds into trays in the high tunnel, we were taking inventory, walking the six acres of fields, planning and mapping out our crops and marketing. We saw dozens of eagles nesting on the bluffs and took time to be naturalists, exploring our surroundings. The first couple of months went by so quickly; we were commuting an hour to work each day until the rental house was ready. We were spending roughly eight to ten hours a day at the farm.

Eric built a sensory table for our son. He has always been perfectly content to play with a handful of toys and a pile of sand or mud. Like any other American child, he has gone through the phases of consumerism and jumped from one childhood icon to another. Luckily, I can still get him to help out, eat healthy and find comfort in nature.

In addition to planting thousands of seeds, our time at La Vista has incubated an immense amount of personal growth. We were welcomed by an outstanding group of community members with open arms, compassionate hearts and a loyal dedication to sustainability. La Vista has felt like home to us since day one. We are grateful daily for the opportunity to work on such a beautiful plot of land complete with breathtaking views, rich biodiversity, perfect prairies and enchanted forests.

Learning how to farm is a complex art. There are always individuals who help guide the process along the way. We have been very fortunate to learn from seasoned farmers who are our mentors and friends. The first farmer at La Vista was Amy Cloud, now co-owner with her husband, Segue Lara, of Three Rivers Community Farm in Elsah, IL. Kris and Stacey Larson, the second farmers, now own Riverbend Roots Farm in Alton, IL. They laid a pretty impressive framework for seed orders, planting dates, field plantings, insect management, soil health and much more. Amy was kind enough to give us a pretty extensive Excel file of planting guides and charts, seed and equipment ordering and much more. Following in their footsteps was no easy undertaking, as they have a plethora of knowledge and experience in sustainable farming. We are very appreciative of our great friendships with the other farmers in our region. It is very important to be a part of an alliance of growers. Having a support system in place to discuss challenges and brainstorm solutions is certainly a must in the vast world of vegetable growing.

Note: The following contains excerpts from an article that was published in the May/June 2014 Issue of GRIT magazine.

We are well into our fifth season as farmers at La Vista CSA Farm on the scenic bluffs overlooking the Mighty Mississippi, the fourth longest river in the world. Where fertile soil meets changing seasons, our journey thus far has been overflowing with a true sense of community, ambition, growth, gratitude, patience and beauty. We have learned more about ourselves, our connection to others and our connection to food than we could have ever imagined. We have been met with many challenges and have learned through trial by fire how to overcome them, to appreciate the art of being humbled and to learn from each season how to improve the next. There is always an underlying current of the precariousness of the elements. Obviously, following a planting calendar according to your zone is a key component to a successful growing year. Luckily, we were given the holy grail of planting charts by the previous farmers of La Vista.

What we have learned is that organic farming is never an exact science. It often weighs heavy on our hearts. Fortunately, we were immediately welcomed into the La Vista community with love, fortitude and support.

We have built friendships that will last a lifetime. Our life at La Vista is wonderful. Growing food for others is our privilege. We are offering seasonal, fresh produce grown with love and without the use of harmful pesticides.

Our connection to the land has become stronger with each changing season. For us, finding the rhythms with the natural calendar is important in knowing when and what to plant. Noticing the annual milestones in your natural surroundings is very important. From a 12-inch square in your own backyard to the stunning acreage that surrounds your garden or farm, it is important to notice which plants are thriving, blooming, fruiting, ripening, working in symbiosis and going to seed, as well as what animals are eating them. Paying attention to these natural rhythms can give so much insight into plant life cycles, knowledge that is a very special part of forming and deepening the connection we have to our food.

There are several milestones, one part intuitive and one part learned, in a calendar year that we rely on to plan, plant, transplant and harvest. Please note these are based on planning and planting in the Midwest (ZONE 6B). You will very quickly know what can grow in your area at any given time by following your local zone-specific planting chart.

Winter Solstice (December 21)

Dormancy — a time of rest and revitalization, the roots holding firmly to the layers of Earth and bedrock beneath; the ground is rich and alive beneath our feet; nutrients are being absorbed from debris and decomposition. The leaves are dormant, but the roots are steadfast with the seasons of change.

The winter solstice marks a good time of year to start thinking ahead and planning for spring.

- Browse through seed catalogs and purchase seeds that will do well in your zone.
- Make wish lists.
- Draw out your garden maps.
- Make a list of materials to acquire.
- Accomplish personal goals before the busy garden season begins.
- Spend more time in nature this year.
- Do more nature-inspired art.

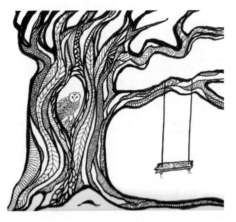

The changing seasons not only astonish me, but always bring about marvel and amazement within my children. I love the way the beauty of the natural world creates a blank canvas for artistic endeavors, an endless supply of materials for mandalas and mobiles, and plenty of "bonding in nature" moments for my family and me. Having an innate love for nature brings so much creativity to life throughout any given season. The colorful array of bountiful produce throughout the growing season becomes a true inspiration for art. We also take the time to discover the wonder of nature throughout the changing seasons.

Winter months can be challenging for both parents and children. Everyone gets a case of cabin fever; perhaps it is a lack of fresh air and sunshine. Maybe it has something to do with the shortage of homegrown produce. Whatever the case, children get stir-crazy and seem to acquire a heightened inquisitiveness. I like to keep my little ones busy with nature exploration. Even in colder temperatures, nature walks always manifest into wonderful adventures. It is amazing to witness imagination coming to life at such an early age.

My daughter helped to make her first nature mandala a few days after she learned how to walk at just 13 months of age. Children are full of artistic expression, and nature allows a platform for originality and a plethora of free colorful materials. While it was Andy Goldsworthy who won the world over with his profound nature creations, art made from or inspired

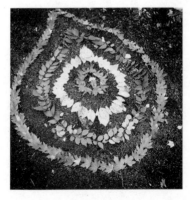

by natural materials can be traced back to the dawn of human civilization. We are wired with creativity. Plants are so versatile in their interconnectedness with us. Not only do they provide absolute beauty for us to gaze upon and profound subject matter for art, but they provide paper for us to write upon, clothes to keep us warm, houses to keep us sheltered and, most importantly, food to sustain us with a delicious and complex array of flavors that are packed with nutrients.

New Year's Day

New Year's Day is composed of equal parts refection and resolution.

Walking from our home (the hermitage) down the tree-lined road that leads to La Vista reveals snow-covered fields from the farm on the right and dozens of eagles soaring above over the course of an hour. Getting lost in the breathtaking landscape almost allows me to take my mind off farmer frustrations such as:

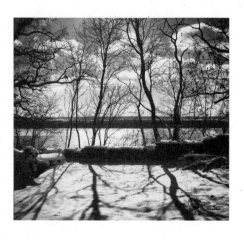

* Dreams of a society that values safe and healthy food languish as I hear more bad news daily in regards to GMOs, food security, laws governing the right to grow, more changes to amendments in our constitution that favor big agriculture.
* Should haves, could haves and would haves about the previous season.

These reflections help to fuel the drive behind our resolutions:

* Focus on the future of food instead of dwelling on the past or sulking in the present.
* Teach more individuals, especially children, how to grow their own food.
* Grow more cover crops.
* Feed the soil more nutrients.
* Till less.
* Integrate more permaculture techniques into our farming practice.
* Plant more flowers for pollinators.

Valentine's Day

On the self-proclaimed most romantic day of the year, you can find my husband and me on our hot date in the greenhouse (hot house), planting thousands of seeds by hand, pouring love from heart to soil as it becomes a form of meditation for us, saying a mantra of intention for each seed, such as: "Grow and thrive little seed. Thank you for nourishing and sustaining us." We find ourselves enthralled in the repetitive motion of sowing seeds. It's a joy to stretch every so often and look up into the sky, where rivers of blackbirds seem to fly for miles.

When the ground begins to thaw and the chill of winter lifts slightly from the fields, my husband begins to till the soil, adding compost and nutrients each step of the way. He sows the first seeds while still able to see his breath in the air. He begins with hardy greens, follows with root crops such as carrots, beets and turnips, then plants peas and gourmet lettuce blends. He tills again in the weeks to follow.

St. Patrick's Day

Each St. Patrick's Day, I have envisioned a "dress like a leprechaun potato-planting party," but it seems as though I am the only one enthusiastic enough about the concept to actually follow through with the comical act.

At any rate, seed potatoes can be planted, and cabbage starts can be transplanted into the fields around March 17 of each year in the Midwest.

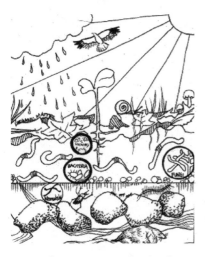

The Vernal Equinox

The vernal equinox, when days and nights are of equal length and the sun rises and sets due east and due west, we like to celebrate by planting seeds in honor of spring. As the celestial equator and the ecliptic intersect, we love to get down close to the earth and witness the emerging beauty of plants as they awaken from the damp rich soil that has been lying dormant in the stillness of winter. As the budding shades of green and white make their way through the cold dark layers, the sun's rays shine down so delicately onto their new growth in such a naturally calculated manner. It is a beautiful time of year to get down close to the earth, in any little square foot of green space, and witness the tiny little microhabitats come to life. Welcome spring! March in the Midwest marks the vernal equinox: the turning point when warmer weather and longer days are on the horizon. The weather can be quite precarious in this region — warm and sunny, rain for days on end, or three feet of snow have all been seen. Typically from late February to early March, the layers of frozen soil begin to thaw, allowing the first green of the season to blanket the soil. In the bitter cold winter, the roots knew when to grab hold of the bedrock below. The plants have intuition. They know when to sprout, where to set roots, when to flower, when to go to seed and when to go dormant. Their life cycles are in tune with the rhythms of nature, the relationship of the Earth to the sun, the soil temperature and the changing seasons. These plants have adapted over thousands of years.

At the vernal equinox, the sun starts to shine long enough for seeds to sprout quickly in the kitchen window. (So fear not if you do not have a greenhouse!) By then, the greenhouse seedlings have grown to their full potential in the inch-wide cell packs they were planted in a month earlier. We hop on the back of the waterwheel transplanter and push the bare roots of each healthy plug into the exposed earth just after the transplanter creates a hole filled with water. Quickly and efficiently, an apprentice and I cover each plug with soil, ensuring its roots are secure in the soil, as my husband idles along on the tractor, straddling each tilled row. We waterwheel-transplant cool-season crops such as cabbage, broccoli, cauliflower, kale, rainbow chard, scallions and head lettuce.

With each passing day, there are farm chores to be done: organizing the outbuildings, sharpening the tools, placing additional seed orders, maintaining the plants in the fields, watering, hand weeding, cultivating, propagating perennials, filling more trays with soil. Our days are long and filled with responsibilities. Our lists get longer as the seasons progress.

After a long and dormant river city winter, the freshness of spring proves a boon for locavores. Chefs, patrons and purveyors have long awaited the farmer's first harvest, whose fields of colorful greens resemble patchwork quilts this time of year.

Greens are among the first crops to emerge. There is something about harvesting greens just after the sun kisses the horizon when the smell of dew is still in the air that is unmatched. Much respect to those who grow greens year-round in high tunnels, cold frames and even indoors, aeroponics- and aquaponics-style. That's true dedication.

A sought-after salad mix revered by growers and chefs alike is composed of vibrant colors, varying textures and layers of flavor. The highly nutritious benefit of spring greens grown without pesticides certainly adds to their charm. While most restaurants offer a deluge of salads made with iceberg and romaine, they pale in comparison to the gorgeous local greens available in the spring and fall in the Midwest. The adventurous palate prefers a salad rich with vibrant lettuces, as well as a diverse array of flavors such as tangy arugula rounded out by the nuttiness of tender young spinach and baby kale. For an even zestier salad blend, spicy Asian mustard greens are peppered into the mix. Ruby Streaks Purple Mustard, Southern Frills, Osaka Purple

Mustard and Tatsoi offer a unique component to any salad. Wild greens such as chickweed and lamb's quarters can be foraged (properly and safely) and added to the mix.

A few tips on planting your own vibrant greens: choose an area in your yard that gets full sun. When the ground thaws in early spring, use a hoe or pitchfork to loosen soil. Sprinkle a few lettuce packs of your choice on the loose soil for mixed greens; plant seeds in rows for heads. Follow seed packet directions for specifics. Sprinkle a shallow layer of soil over the seeds to cover them. Water. Weed. Feed. Harvest. Repeat. Greens are best harvested in the morning before the sun reaches them. Dunk greens in a cool water bath and dry in a salad spinner. Store in a bowl covered with a wet paper towel. Use fresh greens within a few days. Get your green thumb on or be on the lookout for vibrant greens at your area farmers' market.

Before our farm season begins, we offer a preseason share of gourmet salad greens. We cut these greens in the early morning in the humid high tunnel. This is a tedious and often relentless task, but knowing that children and adults are getting the nutrients from the greens into their bodies the very same day we harvest them motivates us to keep on cutting, leaf by leaf, our beautiful blend of lettuce, baby kale, baby spinach and the occasional piece of chickweed that sneaks into our bins. We often don't remove the chickweed because of its wonderful nutrient and mineral content. Watching our children eat greens right from the beds like bunnies is so rewarding, knowing that they are eating healthy, vibrant and nutritious produce grown without pesticides. The astonishing evolution from seed to table is incessantly occurring right before their eyes. They are continuously and instinctively learning where their food comes from, how it is grown and even how to grow it themselves, a skill vital to human existence. Consciously, unconsciously, subconsciously and subliminally, these experiences are being absorbed into their little minds, sculpting them, and will surely have an impact on their lives and their future endeavors.

May

Mid-May marks the transitional period for our farm and others across the Midwest. Our shareholders begin to pick up their weekly share of seasonal vegetables that includes cool-weather crops harvested that morning. Unless you are an avid gardener, you can't get much fresher than that.

Our days are consumed by harvest once our share season begins. It's always surprising just how long harvesting takes. It could take up to two hours to harvest our numbers for the day for just one crop, such as a bunch of baby turnips. We remove the yellow leaves and ones with bug holes in the field prior to taking them to the processing shed to be washed in ice-cold water baths. In one late spring day, a typical harvest would consist of scallions, kale, chard, head lettuce, gourmet lettuce mix, spinach, bunched baby carrots, baby beets and baby turnips, as well as fresh herbs, all multiplied by 60 shares. By the time we harvest, transport to the processing barn, wash, remove outer yellowing leaves, bunch items and set up the share room, the day has disappeared. On share pick-up days, we normally work 12 to 14 hours. Our schedule, aside from harvest days in rain, sleet or shine, is often determined by the weather. If no rain is forecast, we till and plant. If it is raining, we work in the greenhouse. We schedule volunteer workdays to accomplish huge tasks such as harvesting and curing garlic. We rely heavily on them throughout the season; they are vital to accomplishing farm duties.

Each year, Mother's Day brings about the warmer daytime and evening temperatures, making it safe to transplant warm-season crops such as tomatoes, peppers, eggplant, squash, cucumbers and other heat-loving plants. We also direct-seed you-pick crops such as green beans, flowers and heat-loving herbs.

Memorial Day marks the time to start cool-weather crops for fall. We often just repeat the same crops we planted in the spring but change some seeds from early to late varieties. Instead of starting seeds in the greenhouse, we start them on tables under shade trees. They germinate beautifully. Late spring brings on a fluid, seamless rhythm that does not end until late November. Non-stop momentum is another way to describe it.

The Blossoms and Fruit of May

(Previously published in *Feast Magazine*)
The long-anticipated fruits and blossoms in mid-spring are divine. They are vibrant and stunning against the rich backdrop of the diverse hues of greens emerging throughout May. Take notice of the plants growing and blooming beneath your feet in your own backyard or neighborhood park. Humans and plants are in continuous symbiosis. Plants are filled with mystery and wonder. Both their beauty and their nourishment sustain us. Look closely at their intricate patterns, vivid colors and perfect shapes. Breathe in their delicate aromas and savor their complex tastes. Without plants and pollinators, our plates would be empty. All plants have purpose.

Dandelions are notorious for their dual image: their curious negative stereotype as a pesky weed and their whimsical iconic representation of their ability to make wishes come true. Dandelions are actually highly medicinal and are among the most revered plants by herbalists because of their powerful antioxidant and bitter tonic properties. Their greens are best used when tender in the spring and loaded with vitamins and minerals. When young, they are slightly bitter, which gets stronger and less palatable with age. Their flowers are an excellent source of vitamin C, beta-carotene and iron. They have a very unique (sweet + bitter + nutty) flavor and a complex and remarkable texture, in a "wow I'm eating a flower" kind of way. Dandelions can be harvested from areas that are not sprayed with pesticides. Simply pluck the flower from its stem and wash before eating.

Strawberries are at their peak freshness and flavor this time of year. Dainty white blossoms are in full bloom as the sun warms the soil. The fruit actually forms from the blossom, a simple yet miraculous transformation. A time-lapse video of how a strawberry grows will leave any lover of the fruit both humbled and amazed. These ruby gems of the field define the very essence of the first true taste of spring, best picked when fully red. There is nothing quite like biting into a juicy, red vine-ripened strawberry.

Blossoms and fruits pair perfectly together in salads and desserts. Aesthetically, they make an attractive garnish for any dish and are absolutely gorgeous in a refreshing herbal infusion. See Chapter Thirteen.

For backyard garden enthusiasts and farmers, seeing squash blossoms is a sure sign of a forthcoming bountiful harvest. The sunshine-colored blossom emerges first, followed by the long cylindrical zucchini, which is available in almost every shade of green. Summer squash often have a crooked appearance and are found in many shades of yellow. Zucchini squash and summer squash both have the reputation of being some the most prolific crops in the garden. They are even known to produce overnight once the plant is established. One of my favorite varieties is the zephyr squash, a half-green and half-yellow variety of summer squash. It can be purchased online from Johnny's Selected Seeds. Golden zucchini are another personal favorite. We prefer to grow bush varieties rather than vining varieties because they are easier to maintain and harvest. Zucchini are notorious for their rapid growth. They can grow up to 2½ feet long, resembling a caveman's bat. There are thousands of ways to prepare zucchini and squash. While the larger ones can feed a crowd or make a dozen loaves of zucchini bread, it becomes a little tougher and dries out the larger it grows. The most desirable size is between 3 and 6 inches when they are tender yet crisp and richer in flavor. The best way to maintain a crop of tender squash is to harvest daily.

Summer Solstice (June 21)

By the summer solstice, the temperatures often stay in the '80s, '90s and reach up to 110 degrees. Cool-season crops bite the dust. We till the ground and make way for second and third successions and some new varieties of existing crops. Crops planted in midsummer must be planted in the early morning and require drip irrigation to keep them alive in the brutal summer sun. Each summer we have experienced a drought that has lasted up to 48 days. Needless to say, our water bill skyrockets with each drought. Last year was rough for all of the farms in the Midwest. Miraculously, our only crop failures were a shortage of squash in the summer and butternut squash in the fall. We were highly disappointed. However, we exceeded the weekly average value of 22 dollars each and every week during the drought. We were able to offer a plethora of bell peppers, eight pounds of tomatoes, sweet potatoes, Yukon gold and red potatoes, scallions, root vegetables and plenty of fresh herbs, even through the 100-degree weather, which seemed to go on for weeks.

This is the reason we grow a wide array of crops, to ensure that, even in times of drought, members are sure to get the full value of their share each week in the form of several drought-tolerant crops. Our nemeses are insects — thousands and thousands of relentless squash bugs, cucumber beetles, potato beetles, borers, cutworms and aphids that swarm our crops throughout the year. We don't spray pesticides, so we rely on row covers, crop rotation and occasional organic applications such as PyGanic. Nothing solves the problem fully, so we often have to just trust that our shareholders find comfort in a few bug holes here and there, knowing that there were no harmful or toxic chemicals sprayed on their vegetables.

July

The 4th of July typically marks when garlic is ready to be harvested in the Midwest. A good indicator is that the scapes are emerging but are not fully open (in mid- to late June). For a larger garlic bulb, cut the scapes as soon as they surface. Use them to make pesto. See page 146.

To harvest bulbs, tug the stalk gently out of the ground with both hands from the base of the plant. Peel the outer dirt layer and hang in a cool dry area until they have cured, two to three weeks. This process allows the volatile oils to go into the bulbs.

Pulling garlic is one of my favorite tasks on the farm. It is such a rewarding feeling to pull these perfect bulbs after it has taken half the year for them to produce. The smell is overwhelming — for me, in a good way, because I cherish garlic. It is one of the most highly nutritious plants on the planet, and I love everything about it, including its smell.

July is also the season to harvest potatoes, which are best collected using a potato fork. Pressing the fork down into the soil and turning the plant under to expose them feels like finding a treasure. Potatoes are extremely nutritious and very delightful to eat. One important piece of gardening knowledge we learned is that you should never plant tomatoes where potatoes grew the previous year because a deadly late blight might still be in the soil and affect the newly planted tomatoes. They are both in the Solanaceae family, and it is best to follow crop rotations and not plant the same crop or family of crop in the same location.

August

August just might be the hottest month of the year in the Midwest. Don't let that deter you from planting a fall garden. Although most fall crops are started from seed in May, June and July, there is still time to have fresh homegrown produce for fall. In August, if you haven't already started seeds for fall, it is best to buy established plant starts. Most nurseries around town sell plant starts for fall gardening, such as tomatoes, peppers, scallions, squash, cucumber, broccoli, cabbage, kale, chard, lettuce, spinach and pumpkins.

Spinach, kale, chard and lettuce do well when planted now from seed for fall. Plant root crops such as carrots, beets and turnips now for a late fall harvest. Radishes planted now are typically ready to harvest in 30 days. Annual herbs can still be planted to enjoy in late summer/early fall: parsley (actually a biennial), cilantro, basil and dill. Perennial herbs can also be planted now.

Because of the hot weather in August, be sure to either use drip irrigation or water regularly. Pallets make excellent garden beds, and straw bales work well to mulch vegetable crops. Sheet mulch your fall garden for best results.

Compost is a gardener's best friend! A simple compost bin can be made using reclaimed materials such as pallets or an old wire fence panel.

Tomato Season

While we all crave the incomparable flavor of vine-ripened homegrown tomatoes, the plants take a very long time to produce. In midsummer, they need several continuous solid weeks of sunny 90+ degree days in order to ripen. If you just can't wait, blushing tomatoes will ripen in a brown paper bag within a few days. Tape the bag to keep fruit flies out, leave it on the countertop and check daily.

With the green tomatoes, try them fried or in new recipes such as fire-roasted green tomato salsa, green tomato cake or pie or green tomato chutney.

In August, the field heat seems to permeate every cell of my being, making the thick humid air hard to breathe. Being a farmer requires diligence, precision and efficiency as well as long hours, back-breaking labor and intense days in rain, sleet or sun, not to mention an incredibly strong work ethic. Harvesting tomatoes in 110-degree heat with red itchy arms caused by the oils in the tomato leaves, while being swarmed by mosquitoes and bitten by flies, often takes the romance out of organic farming. But, we love what we do. It comes naturally to us. The benefits always outweigh the tribulations at the end of each season.

During this heat, I find solace in the early morning shifts. Before the sun kisses the horizon, I arrive in the fields with my headlamp on and a dozen harvest bins, harvest knife in one hand and high-octane coffee in the other. The peace I find in the fields at this hour cannot be replicated. I can smell the dew still heavy on the plants. I can hear the cardinals and the red-winged blackbirds chirping. I feel so connected and grounded at this hour that I imagine witnessing the plants grow, sinking their roots into the ground further with each passing moment, stretching their stems higher as the sun begins to rise.

Each treacherous summer, we begin to question our dedication to growing at a scale that seems impossible with just a handful of farm workers. We yearn for a future that requires fewer than 80-hour work weeks and toiling in harsh weather. It seems that it's always after an 80-hour work week of 100-degree days that a shareholder throws a complaint on the stack of cinderblocks already heavy on our shoulders. Most complaints come from folks who have never gardened, so they don't understand why "salad things" don't grow at the same time in the Midwest. Even despite their lack of knowledge and our gentle approach to educating them, we take their complaints to heart. As unhealthy as it may be, it's hard not to take them personally, especially after dedicating our waking hours to the farm for months on end and pouring our heart and soul into keeping the plants alive. The complaints get balanced out with compliments. We absolutely love those individuals who show gratitude and empathy. They brighten our days and make it all worthwhile. Gratitude has a beautiful way of turning inches into miles in any given situation.

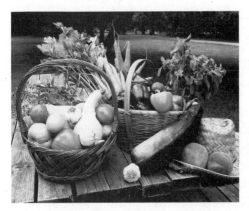

Autumn Equinox

The autumn equinox brings rejuvenation with cooler temperatures and shorter days. Awaking to the crisp, cool autumn air is such a liberating feeling after months of thick air and humidity. The equinox in late September sends a signal to the backyard gardener's cerebral cortex, gently reminding us that it is harvest season and time to be preserving and putting up food for the winter. Within just a couple of short months, the garden will once again become dormant and barren for the year, giving the soil a time to rest. An avid gardener's greatest bounty occurs at this time of year. The seasoned homesteaders and canners have it down to a science, putting up multiple jars of canned tomatoes, sauces, salsas, fruits, vegetables, jams and jellies. Hats off to those folks. Becoming skilled in this age-old hobby requires knowledge of safety measures and temperature regulation as well as time and patience. For first-time canners, taking a few classes through your local extension office before delving into the science of food preservation might be a good idea. I tend to stick to hot water-bath canning and freezing.

In the Midwest, we are fortunate enough to experience all four of the breathtaking seasons. Autumn is especially beautiful in this region. The vibrant colors of rustling leaves in the autumn air are striking and inspiring. The season offers not only a bountiful harvest, but also an abundance of art materials directly from nature, from the beautiful array of fallen leaves to the dried seed pods lying beneath trees, in your own backyard, in nearby parks, on forest floors or on nature trails.

Embrace the nostalgic feelings evoked by each of the changing seasons. Recreate positive memories and start new or renew old traditions with the seasonal landmarks: Spring Equinox (March 20), Summer Solstice (June 21), Autumn Equinox (September 22), Winter Solstice (December 21).

The seasons seem to change in the blink of an eye. Happy autumn! Here are some ideas to savor the season of fall:

* Create nature mandalas with colorful leaves. It is very rewarding and fulfilling as a solo meditation but can be fun with a group of friends or family. Nature mandala walks are also enjoyable. Create them on a day when the

air is still or use small stones to weigh down the leaves. Construct words, patterns or abstract designs with leaves and pods.

* Create window boxes using reclaimed wood. Make as many dividers as you would like. Fill them with things you find on a nature walk that remind you of fall.
* Designate a "seasons" table in your home. Whether it be decorative or educational, collect items found in nature and artistically display them on your table with each changing season.
* Create seasonal living terrariums in fishbowls, large Mason jars or glass containers. Add soil, moss, plants and rocks or geodes. Spray the terrarium twice per week with water and witness the changes in the tiny ecosystem.

October

October typically marks the beginning of the bountiful autumn harvests in the Midwest. Colorful summer bumper crops such as tomatoes, peppers and squash are still producing until mid-October, which marks this region's first frost date. Simultaneously, fall crops such as broccoli, cabbage, winter squash and sweet potatoes are ready to be harvested after their long-awaited seed-to-table journey. Fall greens have emerged from the soil and are abundant again after their summer hiatus.

In October, we plant the final seeds of the year, a bittersweet moment. Early in the month, we plant salad mix, lettuces, spinach, onions, leeks, carrots, herbs, cover crops and bulbs, hoping that some will produce before winter (with the help of row covers) and that some will overwinter for an early spring harvest, assuming that we will have a mild winter. Late fall plantings are always a gamble.

Garlic bulbs (heads of garlic) can be broken apart and the unpeeled individual cloves planted in prepared loose soil in late October for harvesting next July. Simply place them flat side down in small furrows 6 to 8 inches apart. Slightly cover with soil so that you can still see the tips. Mulch the entire patch heavily with straw (a layer 6 to 10 inches thick) to suppress the weeds; the garlic stalk will emerge through the straw in the spring.

The farmer's table is always overflowing with beautiful seasonal dishes literally crafted from field to fork. See the index for recipes.

Cornucopia: Horn of Plenty

According to *Encyclopedia Britannica*, the word "cornucopia" is derived from the Latin *cornu copiae*, meaning "horn of plenty." The cornucopia, revered as

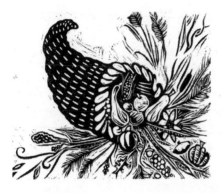

a symbol of bounty or abundance, is typically described as a curled horn of a ram or goat that is packed with the season's harvest. Although the cornucopia is emblematic of the bountiful harvest of the North American Thanksgiving holiday, it can actually be traced back to classical antiquity. Many explanations of its origin and symbolism can be found in Greek mythology, involving Zeus and Hercules, as well as Demeter, the goddess of the Harvest. In one anecdote, Zeus as an infant was nursed and nourished by Almathea, a she-goat. Another mentions that he created the horn of plenty to repay her for nourishing him.

The cornucopia symbolizes an abundant harvest for farmers, the autumn bounty overflowing from our fields to our tables. In the Mississippi River Valley region, the fields of rich dark earth are alive with nutrients, continuously providing nourishment to us. It is truly a time of gratitude. Thanksgiving for us marks the time to glean from the fields. We harvest every last crop and make a huge donation to the nearby food pantry.

As the production and harvesting come to an end, I reflect on the entire season and how it always seems to go by so fast. It takes a great deal of effort to sustain such an operation, and it would not be possible without supporters of the local foods movement. From members to volunteers, small farms rely heavily on community involvement. By the end of each season, I have so much gratitude for members of the farm, assistants, apprentices and volunteers who dedicated so much time, energy and resources into helping the farm thrive.

I invite you to reflect on the positive ways in which your garden, farm or farmer, or even simply the food you have eaten, has affected your life throughout the season. Has the bounty of your harvest fulfilled your healthy lifestyle or your culinary passion? Think of all the people in your life that you have fed with the farm-fresh, sustainably grown vegetables this season. Think of all the individuals you have inspired to try new things or become a little healthier, or the children you have exposed to the beauty of the seed-to-table process.

With immense gratitude and sore bodies, we are excited to take a break from farming after this season. We wish to scale down, focus on permaculture and soil building and begin an eco-retreat center which will house resilient living workshops, educational seminars and lots of gardening projects.

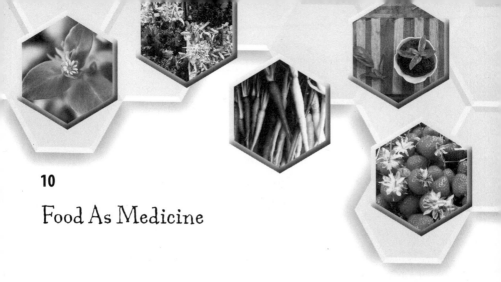

10

Food As Medicine

Let food be thy medicine and medicine be thy food.

— Hippocrates

IMPROVING YOUR PHYSICAL WELL-BEING by living a healthy lifestyle is a lifelong process. Contrary to what many people believe, health does not have to be complicated. By making small changes over time and focusing on long-term health over short-term success, you can make a world of difference. The most important things to remember are that whole, unprocessed foods are like nature's gift to your health and that daily movement is one of the best ways to improve blood circulation, boost the immune system, reduce stress and symptoms of depression, and raise overall levels of happiness and satisfaction. Mental health and physical health are two sides of the same coin, and you must address both to be truly, wholly healthy.

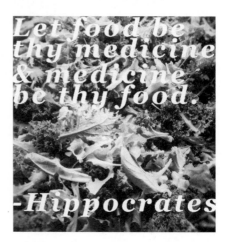

What We Put into Our Bodies Has the Potential to Heal Us or Impair Us

Lifestyle changes for optimal health:

* Drink more water.
* Get plenty of fresh air and sunshine.
* Spend time with loved ones and those who uplift you.

* Laughter induces happiness. Surround yourself with things that make you smile.
* Self-love is crucial in overall health and well-being. Self-love can come in many forms: quiet time to meditate, reflect or do yoga, morning smoothies, juicing, gardening, taking time out of your busy life to focus on things that bring you happiness.
* Exercising and spending time outside improve overall health and well-being. Hike, walk, run, jog or dance regularly.
* Try to incorporate contemplative practices into your life, such as meditation, yoga, qigong or tai chi.
* Reduce stress by engaging in activities you love on a regular basis. If you don't already have one, find a hobby that you can practice on a weekly basis.
* Maintain a garden! Studies have shown that gardening actually makes you happier because touching the soil with your bare hands increases your dopamine levels.
* Stop smoking. According to the Centers for Disease Control, smoking has been attributed to one in five deaths each year in the US alone. Smoking increases your risk of cancer, COPD, coronary heart disease and stroke. Smoking reduces overall health and affects nearly every organ in the body from the skin, teeth and hair to the lungs and cardiovascular and reproductive systems.
* Saturated fats, polyunsaturated fats, trans fats: According to the CDC, these unhealthy fats can increase the bad cholesterol LDL in your bloodstream, which in turn increases risk of coronary heart disease. They also decrease the good cholesterol HDL.
* Consider seasonal colon cleanses. If you have a poor diet or lots of stress, a seasonal colon cleanse might help improve digestion and increase energy levels. Start by eating a healthy diet for a few days — ancient grains, good fats, fresh raw fruits and vegetables and lots of water. Slowly eliminate cooked foods for a few days and try to eat raw. Follow that with a juice fast for one to three days. Slowly integrate fresh fruits and vegetables into your diet and gradually add cooked foods. Seasonal cleanses are meant to detoxify the liver and to clear unwanted buildup from the digestive tract. Colonics treatments are useful if you are continuously experiencing digestion issues. Consult your doctor to see if a colon cleanse, juice fast or colonics treatment would be right for you, based on your medical history.

Slowly removing the following bad stuff from your diet can lead to over-all health improvement:

* Refined sugar: Sugar lowers the immune system, disrupts the glucose balance in the body, raises blood pressure and increases your risk of diabetes and coronary disease.
* Artificial sweeteners: Just because many of these substances are calorie-free does not mean they are healthy. They disrupt the chemical balance in your body and encourage weight gain, mental cloudiness and other health issues.
* Processed foods: These over-packaged, over-processed foods contain high amounts of preservatives, artificial colors and flavorings, saturated and trans fats, sugar and salt.
* Soda: One 12-ounce can of soda contains approximately eight teaspoons of sugar.
* Pesticides and herbicides: These agricultural chemicals are harmful to our health and to the environment. They have been linked to cancer and other life-threatening illnesses. They have also been known to inhibit hormones.
* Ingredients you cannot pronounce: This is a good rule of thumb for avoiding unnecessary synthetic additions in your food.
* Excessive caffeine intake: According to the Mayo Clinic, an amount over 500–600 mg per day of caffeine can lead to insomnia, nervousness, irritability, stomach problems, increased heart rate and muscle tremors.

Try to incorporate the following small changes in your diet over time:

* Certified organic coconut oil
* Butter rather than margarine
* Organic and free-range eggs
* Maple syrup, honey, liquid stevia extract or dates instead of refined sugar
* Plenty of raw fruits, vegetables and garlic
* Lots of fresh herbs such as cilantro, parsley, sage and rosemary
* A natural daily fiber supplement such as ground flax seeds, flax oil or flax meal
* Probiotics instead of antibiotics
* Fermented foods such as sauerkraut, kimchi, kefir, kombucha, miso and pickles

Food As Medicine: Grow and Eat These Highly Nutritious Vegetables

All vegetables and fruits have nutritional content, but some are more nutrient-dense. The most important thing is to vary your diet to obtain a full

spectrum of nutrients from many different whole food sources. It never ceases to amaze me just how many nutrients can be found in plants. This is a
partial list of vegetables that we have grown in the Midwest. Check for what
will grow in your zone.

Asparagus contains nutrients including vitamins A, C, B6 and a significant
amount of folate, a major player in blood cell formation.

Beets help to improve overall liver function and aid in detoxification. They
are high in antioxidants and phytonutrients and contain generous amounts of
potassium, folate, manganese, magnesium and iron.

Broccoli has cancer-prevention and cancer-fighting properties. It also
helps to create enzyme production for digestion.

Brussels sprouts are extremely high in vitamins C and K and have generous
amounts of folate, vitamin B6 and manganese. Like all cruciferous vegetables,
they have wonderful antioxidant properties. Lightly steamed, they have been
known to help lower cholesterol.

Cabbage and cauliflower contain cancer-prevention and cancer-fighting
properties. They help to create enzyme production for digestion.

Celery is rich in phytonutrients, antioxidants, folic acid, minerals and vitamins C, A and K.

Chard, as a protective mechanism for the liver, helps to neutralize metals,
chemicals and pesticides built up in the body and supports the endocrine
system.

Corn contains antioxidant phytonutrients such as beta-carotene. It is a
great source of manganese, B-complex vitamins and fiber.

Garlic, originating in Central Asia, is one of the most healing plants and also
the earliest documented used by humans. The ancient Egyptian, Greek and
Roman civilizations revered garlic as sacred, using it not only for its culinary
charm but also for its highly medicinal properties. It is also mentioned throughout Ayurvedic texts. Garlic, a natural antibiotic, is rich in protein and vitamins
A, B6 and B1 and contains manganese, iron, copper, selenium and calcium. It
is abundant in antioxidants and has antibacterial, antifungal, antimicrobial and
anti-inflammatory properties. Garlic helps to cleanse the liver and flush out
toxins. Its flavor is unforgettable and makes so many dishes more enjoyable.

Preserve peeled garlic cloves in apple cider vinegar and refrigerate the jar.
Use them for easy prep or munch on when cold and flu symptoms begin.

Within the two classifications of garlic, hard-necked and soft-necked,
there are ten separate groups. Soft-necked varieties can easily be made into
garlic braids at harvest time.

Hot peppers, such as chili peppers, contain capsaicin, an active phytochemical that acts as a defense mechanism to deter insects and animals from eating them. With its powerful medicinal properties, it has been used to kill bacteria, fight cancer, relieve headaches, clear congestion, provide topical pain relief, reduce cholesterol and burn fat. Dry hot peppers and add them to your favorite soups and stews all winter long!

Kale acts as a protective mechanism for the liver and helps to neutralize metals, chemicals and pesticides. It contains an astounding amount of vitamins K, C and A as well as copper, which help support the endocrine system.

Kohlrabi, like other cruciferous vegetables, is an excellent source of vitamins C and A; it has tremendous antioxidant properties and is loaded with phytonutrients.

Leeks are rich in vitamins A, K, E and C, folic acid and riboflavin. They also contain antioxidant properties.

Onions are rich in antioxidants and phytochemicals. They also contain vitamin C, manganese and B-complex vitamins.

Potatoes, aside from being a good source for carbohydrates, contain folate, iron, magnesium, calcium and vitamins C, A and K.

Spinach, an excellent source of iron, is high in phytonutrients and loaded with vitamins.

Summer squash contains antioxidant and anti-inflammatory properties. It is high in vitamin C, copper, magnesium and manganese.

Strawberries are loaded with antioxidants and are high in vitamin C and manganese. They also contain anti-inflammatory phytonutrients.

Sweet potatoes are an excellent source of vitamins A, C and B6 as well as copper and manganese. Rich in antioxidants, especially beta-carotene, they also contain anti-inflammatory properties.

Tomatoes are rich in phytonutrients and antioxidants including lycopene and beta-carotene. They are an excellent source of vitamins B, C, E and K, as well as copper, folate, potassium and manganese.

Tomatillos are rich in antioxidant phytochemicals known to have anti-cancer and antibacterial properties.

Winter squash is rich in antioxidants, carotenoids, copper, manganese, potassium and vitamins A, B and C. It is an excellent source of fiber.

Food As Medicine

Food and water are the most basic necessities for survival. Vitamins and minerals that our bodies need to function can be found in fresh fruits and vegetables, legumes, nuts and whole grains. Meat and fish also are major sources of protein, but they are not necessary for survival. In this chapter, we focus on the basic nutritional benefits of fruits, vegetables, legumes, nuts and whole grains, each of which supports the various systems in our bodies.

Skeletal System

The skeletal system offers a framework for the rest of the body. Comprised of 206 bones and over 340 joints, it protects our vital organs, veins, arteries, nerves and muscles.

The following support the skeletal system:

- Calcium (kale, broccoli, mustard greens, dandelion greens, Napa cabbage, okra, arugula, garlic, sun-dried tomatoes, collard greens, turnip greens)
- Magnesium (sweet potatoes, beet greens, spinach, collard greens, tomatoes, okra, potatoes, artichokes, raisins)
- Potassium (bananas, plantains, oranges, papaya, sweet potatoes, spinach, potatoes, tomatoes)
- Vitamin C (green peppers, red peppers, broccoli, Brussels sprouts, oranges, grapefruits, pineapple, papaya)
- Vitamin D (mushrooms)
- Vitamin K (parsley, Brussels sprouts, broccoli and dark leafy greens including kale, spinach, turnip greens, mustard greens, Swiss chard, romaine lettuce)

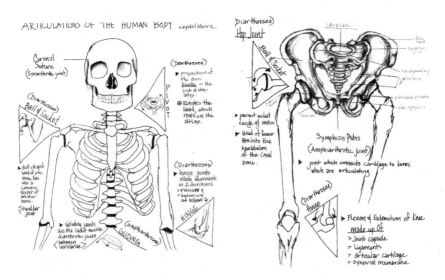

◉ Herbs that support bone and joint health include black cohosh, ginger, turmeric, gingko, red clover.

Central Nervous System

The central nervous system (CNS), the command center of the body, comprises the brain, retina and spinal cord. It controls most of the functions of the mind and the body. The following support the CNS:

◉ Antioxidants (cocoa, blueberries, pomegranates, red wine, garlic)
◉ Vitamin K (dark leafy greens including kale, spinach, turnip greens)
◉ Omega-3 fatty acids (seeds and nuts)
◉ Magnesium and B6 (brown rice, whole grains)
◉ Herbs that support the CNS include kava kava, chamomile, skullcap, lobelia, gingko, black cohosh, hyssop

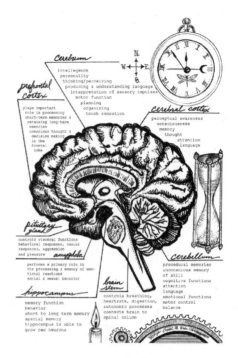

The eyes are the organs of sight that allow light to pass through the cornea, pupil, lens and then retina. The iris is a muscle that controls pupil size and light. It also determines eye color. Electrical impulses are generated by rods and cones (receptors in the retina) and travel through the optic nerve to the brain. The muscles in the eyes are controlled by cranial nerves.

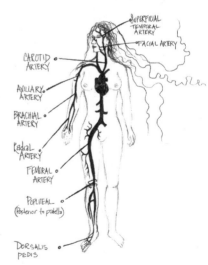

The Circulatory System

The circulatory system transports nutrients, water and oxygen throughout the body's billions of cells. It also helps to flush out carbon dioxide and other waste products produced by cells.

The following support the circulatory system:

- Omega-3 fatty acids (flax seeds, chia seeds, nuts)
- B vitamins (dark leafy greens, parsley, red peppers, beets, broccoli, wild Alaskan salmon)
- Calcium (dark leafy greens, sesame seeds, tofu, cheese). Alternatives are blood cleansers. They assimilate nutrients and eliminate wastes. Plantain, red clover, dandelion, burdock and garlic help cleanse the blood.

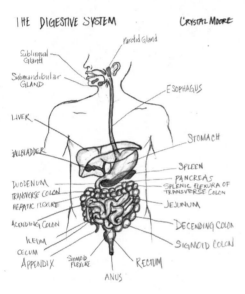

THE DIGESTIVE SYSTEM — CRYSTAL MOORE

Parotid Gland
Sublingual Gland
Submandibular GLAND
LIVER
GALLBLADDER
DUODENUM
TRANSVERSE COLON
HEPATIC FLEXURE
ACENDING COLON
ILEUM
CECUM
APPENDIX
SIGMOID FLEXURE
ANUS
ESOPHAGUS
STOMACH
SPLEEN
PANCREAS
SPLENIC FLEXURA OF TRANSVERSE COLON
JEJUNUM
DECENDING COLON
SIGMOID COLON
RECTUM

Digestive System

The digestive system helps to break food down into smaller molecules of nutrients before being absorbed in the blood and transported to cells throughout the body for nourishment and energy.

The mouth and teeth play huge roles in the body's ability to perform basic functions including digestion, speech and taste. Teeth are vital in chewing food into smaller pieces for swallowing and providing support for the facial muscles. Mucous membranes line and protect the inside of the mouth and keep it wet. The tongue is covered in papillae that host the taste buds. The salivary glands secrete saliva and also contain amylase, a digestive enzyme responsible for breaking down carbohydrates. The orbicularis oris muscle is responsible for the movement of the lips.

The following support the mouth and teeth:

- Fresh fruits and vegetables
- Calcium-rich foods (dark leafy greens, sesame seeds, tofu, cheese, yogurt, almonds)
- Turmeric
- Whole grains
- Foods rich in vitamin C (green peppers, red peppers, broccoli, Brussels sprouts, oranges, grapefruits, pineapple, papaya)

⊕ Herbs and other natural substances to support a healthy mouth and healthy teeth include turmeric powder, tea tree oil, myrrh gum, baking soda, hydrogen peroxide and water rinse, oil pulling (rinsing the mouth with organic coconut oil for a few minutes each day).

Historically, cultures around the world have used healing plants, twigs, stems and roots to care for their mouth and teeth. Twigs containing medicinal properties can be used in lieu of a toothbrush. Eucalyptus, fir and oak all contain volatile oil, tannins and vitamins that promote mouth and teeth health.

Foods that support the digestive system are rich in the following: probiotics and lactic acid (fermented foods, yogurt), fiber (sprouted whole grains, flax) and potassium (bananas). Herbs that support the digestive system include ginger, peppermint, basil, dill and licorice.

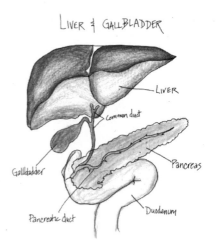

LIVER & GALLBLADDER

LIVER

Common duct

Pancreas

Gallbladder

Pancreatic duct

Duodenum

The liver is responsible for the uptake and storage of nutrients — including fat, proteins and carbohydrates — as well as the disposal of toxins, the production of synthetic proteins critical for blood clotting and the metabolism of substances produced by the body. The gallbladder assists the liver by storing and releasing bile.

Foods that support the liver and gallbladder are rich in the following:

⊕ Omega-3 fatty acids (seeds and nuts)

⊕ Antioxidants found in fruits and vegetables

⊕ Cruciferous vegetables (broccoli, cabbage, kale, collards, turnip greens, bok choi)

⊕ Dark leafy greens help to neutralize metals, pesticides and chemicals and act as a protective mechanism for many organs and body systems

⊕ Turmeric can help detoxify the liver, digest fats and stimulate bile production

⊕ Garlic is a natural antibiotic that helps to boost immunity, fight infection and detoxify the liver

⊕ Beta-carotene (carrots, butternut squash, sweet potatoes)

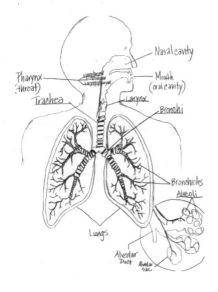

Nasal cavity

Pharynx
(throat)

Mouth
(oral cavity)

Trachea

Larynx

Bronchi

Bronchioles
Alveoli

Lungs

Alveolar
Duct   Alveolar
Sac

🌀 Herbs supporting the liver and gall-bladder include milk thistle, burdock root, dandelion root, peppermint and yellow dock root.

Respiratory System

The respiratory system assists in the exchange of gases between blood and air and also between blood and the body's billions of cells. The organs of the respiratory system help to filter, warm, humidify and distribute oxygen throughout the body. It plays a significant role in our speech and in our sense of smell. It helps the body to maintain homeostasis.

The following support the respiratory system:

🌀 Antioxidant-rich fruits and vegetables
🌀 Cruciferous vegetables (broccoli, cabbage, kale, collards, turnip greens, bok choi)
🌀 Vitamin C (dark leafy greens, citrus)
🌀 Herbs including mullein, astragalus, fennel, fenugreek, sage, parsley, oregano and thyme

Olfactory System

The olfactory system comprises the nose and nostrils, olfactory hairs (or nerve fibers), olfactory bulbs, olfactory cells, as well as specialized nerve cells found throughout the olfactory tracts. Smell is detected through the nostrils and converted into signals throughout the olfactory tract sent through neurons, where the brain can identify smells. This system is closely related to the limbic system, which is responsible for memory and emotions. It is also strongly related to the sense of taste — most of your taste sensation is actually due to smell.

Lymphatic System

The lymphatic system comprises nodes, vessels and capillaries responsible for transporting lymph fluid from tissues to the bloodstream. Lymphatic tissue filters the lymph. This system is also responsible for transporting fatty acids to the circulatory system. It removes toxins from the body, helps to drain excess fluids and distributes nutrients throughout the body.

The following support the lymphatic system:

◉ Potassium-rich foods (bananas, broccoli)
◉ Fresh-squeezed lemon in warm water daily
◉ At least eight glasses of filtered or purified water per day
◉ Herbs including burdock root, calendula flower, cleavers, red clover and mullein

Immune System

The immune system comprises primarily specialized cells, lymphoid tissues, organs and proteins (listed below) that work together to form the body's natural defense system against harmful organisms and invaders. Sugar and processed foods weaken the immune system, making the body more susceptible to disease.

◉ Thymus: Immune develpment until maturity
◉ Liver: Responsible for synthesizing proteins. Specialized cells ingest bacteria in the blood
◉ Bone marrow: Cells involved in the immune system begin their development in the bone marrow
◉ Tonsils: Collections of lymphocytes
◉ Lymphocytes: Produce antibodies
◉ Lymph nodes: Cells communicate with one another in the lymph nodes
◉ Spleen: Filters the blood, organisms and cells of the immune system
◉ Blood: Carries proteins and cells from one section of the body to another

These foods boost immunity:

◉ Garlic
◉ Herbal tea, black tea, green tea
◉ Mushrooms
◉ Oats and barley
◉ Probiotics
◉ Sweet potatoes

Herbs for cold and flu support include:

◉ Cayenne
◉ Echinacea

- Elderberry
- Ginger
- Goldenseal
- Marshmallow
- Oregano
- Sage
- Slippery elm bark
- Thyme

Other natural cold and flu remedies include:

- Honey and lemon
- Honey and cinnamon
- Hot vinegar steam
- Essential oil steam
- Hot herbal bath (peppermint, sage, rosemary)
- Neti pot (used according to package directions)
- Hot toddy
- Salt water gargle (2 tablespoons sea salt dissolved in 1 cup warm water)
- 5 drops of pure eucalyptus oil mixed with ½ cup coconut oil and rubbed on chest and feet
- Oregano oil (used according to directions on label)
- Elderberry syrup
- Horehound cough drops

Endocrine System

The endocrine system is the grid of glands that produces hormones and helps to maintain and regulate body functions. It regulates homeostasis, immunity, reproduction and development.

Metabolism converts the food we eat into energy through a series of chemical reactions that occur in the cells of our body. The enzymes in the digestive system break down proteins to form amino acids. Fats are broken down into fatty acids. Carbohydrates are broken down into simple sugars such as glucose. The compounds are then absorbed into the bloodstream and transported to the cells in the body. Enzymes regulate the chemical reactions engaged in metabolism. These are all ways the body may source energy. Energy is released and can be used or stored in tissues, organs, muscles and fat. The thyroid regulates the body's metabolism with help from the hypo-thalamus and the pituitary gland.

The following support the endocrine system:

- Iodine (sea vegetables, kelp, kombu, seaweed)
- Antioxidants found in fruits and vegetables
- Healthy fats (avocado, chia seeds, sunflower seeds, pumpkin seeds, spirulina)
- Vitamins and minerals (leafy greens, cruciferous vegetables, asparagus)
- Vitamin D (mushrooms, oranges)
- Herbs including adaptogen herbs (used for overall health and wellness), astragalus, holy basil, ginseng, ashwaganda and shisandra

Female Reproductive System

The female reproductive system consists of the female anatomy within the pelvis. It is made up of the vulva, vagina, mons pubis, labia, clitoris, urethra, hymen, uterus, cervix, fallopian tubes and ovaries. The ovaries produce hormones including estrogen and progesterone that regulate many reproductive processes. This system allows a woman to have sexual intercourse, produce ova (eggs), protect and nourish and develop a fertilized egg, house the fetus in the amniotic sac, nourish it with oxygen from the placenta and give birth. When labor begins, oxytocin, a pituitary hormone, causes the walls of the uterus to contract, which leads the cervix to dilate. The afterbirth (placenta) follows the fetus.

Menstruation occurs typically once per month (every 28 days) during ovulation, when an ovary sends an egg into the fallopian tubes. The egg dries up and leaves the body after two weeks unless it is fertilized by sperm. The menstrual flow (blood and tissues from the inner lining of the uterus,) typically lasts for three to seven days. PMS, or premenstrual syndrome, may occur seven days prior to the flow and include symptoms such as fatigue, sore breasts, backaches, irritability, depression and/or difficulty concentrating. Abdominal cramping is common as prostaglandins cause the smooth muscle in the uterus to contract.

The following support the female reproductive system:

- Whole grains
- Fiber-rich foods (beans, fruits, vegetables)
- Iron-rich foods (lentils, spinach, lean meats)

- Antioxidant-rich foods and foods containing beta-carotene (squash, pumpkins, carrots)
- Foods containing folic acid and B vitamins (figs, kale, berries)
- Foods containing calcium, vitamin A and vitamin C (cruciferous vegetables, kale and other dark leafy greens, sprouted nuts)
- Foods containing probiotics (yogurt, kefir, fermented foods)
- Clean and lean protein (pasture-raised meats, sprouted nuts and seeds, farm eggs)
- Herbs including black cohosh, chaste tree berry, dong quai root, ginger, motherwort, red raspberry leaf and red clover

Male Reproductive System

The male reproductive system consists of the reproductive organs (genitals), including the testicles, the duct system made up of the vas deferens and the epididymis, the accessory glands including the prostate gland and the seminal vesicles as well as the penis. In a mature male, the testes produce and house millions of sperm cells. The testicles (which are also part of the endocrine system) produce hormones, mainly testosterone, that cause boys to develop deeper voices as well as body and facial hair during puberty. The function of the male reproductive system is to produce as well as secrete male sex hormones and to produce and maintain sperm. It also is responsible for transporting sperm and semen, which is discharged into the female reproductive tract during intercourse. The penis is also responsible for urination.

The following support the male reproductive system:

- Whole grains
- Lean and clean proteins and vitamin D (pasture-raised meats, sprouted nuts and seeds, lentils, farm eggs)
- Vitamins and minerals from fresh fruits and vegetables
- Foods containing selenium (brown rice, shrimp, Brazil nuts, walnuts, wild Alaskan salmon)
- Herbs including American ginseng, gotu kola, maca root, licorice root, saw palmetto berry, Siberian ginseng, tribulus fruit, yohimbe bark

Kidneys and Urinary Tract

The kidneys and urinary tract filter and eliminate wastes from the blood and regulate the body's balance of water to ensure that its tissues are healthily maintained. The urinary tract consists of the ureters, the bladder and the urethra. The kidneys produce urine, the by-products of metabolism, which include water, salts and toxins. The kidneys also regulate the body's pH levels (acid/base balance of fluids and blood), regulate blood pressure and produce renin, an enzyme that helps to regulate salt levels. The kidneys secrete erythropoietin, a hormone that controls and stimulates red blood cell production.

The following support the kidneys and urinary tract:

- Foods that contain flavonols (berries, especially cranberries)
- Fermented and probiotic-rich foods (fermented foods and beverages, cultured foods, yogurt)
- Garlic
- Foods rich in antioxidants (especially cinnamon, apples, grapes, cacao, grapeseed extract)
- Herbs including goldenrod, stinging nettle leaf and uva ursi

Integumentary System

The integumentary system, consisting of the skin (the largest organ), hair, nails and specialized nerves and glands, reduces water loss. It contains specialized receptors that protect the body, regulate body temperature and respond to touch. This system also protects the body from dehydration and infection, assists in disposing waste materials and stores fat and water.

The following support the integumentary system:

- Vitamin A (butternut squash, carrots, sweet potatoes, lettuce, fish, dark leafy greens)
- Vitamin C (dark leafy greens, citrus)
- Calcium (kale, broccoli, mustard greens, dandelion greens, Napa cabbage, okra, arugula, garlic, sun-dried tomatoes, collard greens, turnip greens)
- Herbs including aloe vera, burdock root, calendula, chickweed, comfrey, plantain, self-heal violet, witch hazel, yarrow

What Makes the Body Go?

Proteins, enzymes, carbohydrates and fats, oh my!

Proteins are built from 16 amino acids and form complex molecular structures. They are crucial in many cell functions, build and repair body tissues, act as antibodies and provide defense against germs. Structural proteins are responsible for movement within the body, as well as structural support.

Enzymes help speed up chemical reactions and begin the breakdown of protein molecules into amino acids in the small intestine. These amino acids are then absorbed into the blood and transported throughout the body to build cell structures.

Carbohydrates provide energy for the body. Simple carbohydrates are just one or two sugar molecules like glucose, lactose and fructose. Complex carbohydrates, also called dietary starch, consist of a long string of sugar molecules. Starches are found in grains and vegetables and often contain a lot of dietary fiber. Simple carbohydrates are found in fruits and sweeteners, and as added sugar in processed foods. The body converts most carbohydrates to glucose to be absorbed into the bloodstream and used by cells for energy. As glucose levels rise, the pancreas releases the hormone insulin, which aids in transporting sugar from the blood into the cells as a source of energy.

Fats are a major source of energy for the body and help to maintain body temperature. Fat-soluble vitamins and minerals are stored in fatty tissue and the liver.

Vitamins function in the processes of digestion, metabolism and immunity. Vitamins are essential for the health of the organs, tissues and cells and help to process proteins, carbohydrates and fats. There are 13 essential vitamins: A, C, D, E, K and the B vitamins, which include biotin, thiamine, folic acid and riboflavin. Most vitamins are obtained through food, especially fresh fruits and vegetables.

Minerals transmit nerve impulses, help build strong bones, regulate the heart and make hormones. Macrominerals consist of calcium, chloride, iron, magnesium, potassium, sodium and sulfur. Trace minerals consist of cobalt, copper, fluoride, iodine, iron, manganese, selenium and zinc.

Essential amino acids come from our food. Animal sources of protein offer all the essential amino acids humans need, but other protein-rich foods combined in a varied diet will also fill our requirements.

Non-meat sources of proteins include avocado, broccoli, kale, spinach, sweet potato, nuts and seeds, grains, legumes and other plant-based foods such as tofu and tempeh. The variety and nutritional offerings of this food group are astounding.

Legumes: Black beans, black-eyed peas, black turtle beans, Boston beans, cannellini beans, chickpeas (garbanzo beans), cranberry beans, Egyptian beans, fava beans, field peas, great Northern beans, green beans, kidney beans, lentils, lespedeza, licorice, Lima beans, Madagascar beans, Mexican black beans, mung beans, mung peas, navy beans, peanuts, peas, Peruvian beans, pinto beans, red beans, red clover, red kidney beans, scarlet runner beans, southern peas, sugar snap peas, soybeans, wax beans

Tofu is soybean curd — choose organic and non-GMO.

Tempeh is fermented soybean curd. Some consider tempeh to be healthier because of the many good bacteria activated through the fermentation process.

True nuts and nut-like drupe seeds (best when soaked and sprouted): almonds, Brazil nuts, cashews, kola nuts, pecans, pistachios, walnuts

Seeds (best when soaked and sprouted): Hemp seeds, sunflower seeds, flax seeds, sesame seeds

Nut and seed butters can be made from most varieties and are excellent sources of protein. My favorites are sunflower, almond and cashew butters and tahini, a butter made from sesame seeds. You can also use nuts and seeds to make dairy-free milks. Hemp, almond and soy milk are the most popular.

Healthy grains include: Amaranth, barley, brown rice, bulgur, wheat, millet, oats, quinoa, wild rice, wheat berries and farro. Sprouted grains and sprouted grain breads are especially good.

Herbal Support

There are many good books that list recommendations for herbal support, along with dosage and the contraindications for each herb. Rosemary Gladstar and Susan Weed are two of my favorite authors on herbal medicine.

Headache support: Cayenne, chamomile, dandelion, feverfew, ginger, gingko leaf, goldenrod, lavender essential oil, lemon balm, licorice, mullein flower, mugwort, osha, passionflower, peppermint, rose petals, sage, skullcap, willow, yarrow

Digestive support: Basil, cilantro, dill, ginger, licorice, peppermint

Mucus membrane support: Comfrey, chickweed, marshmallow, hollyhock, slippery elm

Bleeding and the discharge of mucus support: Yarrow

Soft organic tissue support: Astringent herbs like cranesbill, mullein, red raspberry, witch hazel, yarrow

Fatigue support: St. John's wort, kava kava, ginseng

Cancer Prevention and Support

According to Food Choices for Cancer Prevention and Survival, "More than 1.6 million people are diagnosed with cancer each year in the United

States." Neal Barnard, MD, founder and president of the PCRM (Physicians Committee for Responsible Medicine), founded Food for Life, a "program dedicated to cancer prevention and survival." His prevention methods include consuming more fresh sources of "antioxidants including vitamin C, vitamin E, beta-carotene, selenium, lycopene and others to help neutralize the damaging effects of oxygen in the body, helping to prevent free radicals from attacking cell membranes and potentially causing damage to DNA." Food Choices for Cancer Prevention and Survival can be downloaded free at pcrm.org (http://pcrm.org/sites/default/files/pdfs/health/HealthyEatingForLife.pdf).

Foods suggested for cancer prevention: Grapefruit, berries, sweet potatoes, wild-caught Alaskan salmon, green tea, ground flax seed, cruciferous vegetables (broccoli, cauliflower, cabbage) that contain phytonutrients, turmeric, dark leafy greens

Foods known to kill cancer cells: Broccoli, cauliflower, kale, cabbage, berries, tomatoes, walnuts, garlic, beans

Foods rich in antioxidants: Fruits (grapefruit, apples, oranges, pineapple, strawberries), brassicas (broccoli, cauliflower, cabbage, Brussels sprouts), greens (spinach), vegetables (carrots, sweet potatoes), legumes (chickpeas, beans), brown rice

Superfoods

The term "superfood" tends to be another buzzword thrown around as a marketing strategy, but superfoods actually are beneficial to health. These are some of the healthiest foods on Earth, determined by three key components: antioxidants, nutrients and fiber: Kale, broccoli, beets, pumpkin, leeks, cauliflower, garlic, ginger, blueberries, strawberries, watermelon, apples, cranberries, green tea, wild salmon, Greek yogurt, quinoa, chia, oatmeal, beans, lentils, almonds and pistachios.

Juicing

I have been juicing since 2000, when I started work at the juice bar at Wild Oats, a natural foods market. This gave me a significant benefit: I drank a lot of juice. I would substitute meals with a 24-ounce Earth Goddess (carrots, beets, celery, spinach, parsley and spirulina). I felt a true sense of vitality when juicing regularly. Take advantage of the bountiful season and juice your produce. The benefits are outstanding: maximum nutrition and health, an increase in energy, a sense of mental clarity. Don't have a juicer? Find a friend with a juicer and juice in good company.

Kids love fresh juice. Iris has been drinking it since before she could walk. Carrot juice is a great option for them, with its powerful antioxidants, beta-carotene, vitamins C, A and B and instant energy.

Green smoothies: The one trend that should never go out of style! For a quick, nutritious snack or meal replacement, add two handfuls of dark, leafy greens such as kale or spinach to any smoothie. Our favorite includes frozen banana, frozen pineapple, coconut milk, hemp seeds, kale, spinach, honey and spirulina.

Best practices in a healthy diet:

⊕ Buy locally, know your farmer.
⊕ Choose organic.
⊕ Integrate fermented foods.
⊕ Eat a diet rich in fresh fruits and vegetables.
⊕ Keep a list of superfoods in your wallet to remind you at the market.
⊕ Eat wild foods.
⊕ Have healthy food potlucks with friends and family.
⊕ Grow your own food! Join a CSA!

Note: This chapter was reviewed by Carrie Magill, MD.

create

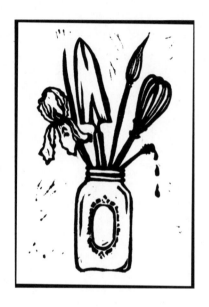

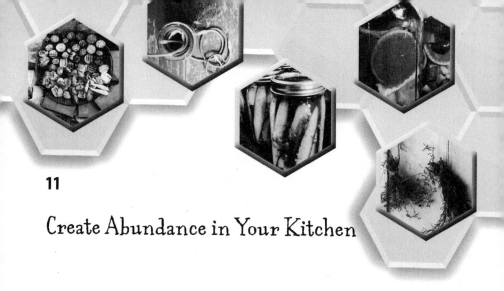

11

Create Abundance in Your Kitchen

Preserving Herbs

P RESERVING HERBS is a good place to start. Take advantage of the plethora of fresh herbs growing in your garden while they are at their prime. Don't miss the chance to preserve that beautiful fresh herb flavor for use in all of your culinary creations through the winter months. Of the many ways to preserve herbs, the most popular might be drying, but making herb butters, herb-infused oils and vinegars and various kinds of pesto are also excellent options.

Herbs are one of those garden glories that often get overlooked during the frenzy of harvest and canning season. Culinary herbs are not only flavorful but, as mentioned in Chapter Three, are very nutritious and often highly medicinal.

During harvest season, display your herbs like a bouquet, in a glass of water, where they will last up to a week. Just pinch some off when you need any. To maximize freshness, change the water each day. You will be surprised how fresh your herbs stay!

Drying Herbs

Either use a food dehydrator or string bundled herbs upside down in a dry place. When the leaves are crisp, remove from stems and store in labeled and dated glass jars. Once you have multiple dried herbs, you can create custom spice blends. Create a handmade label and give as gifts to friends and family.

Freezing Herbs

One of the easiest ways to capture their essence is to simply cut fresh herbs with a pair of scissors and freeze them in ice cube trays. Cut the leaves from stems. Fill ice cube trays with water, and then firmly place herbs (roughly

1 teaspoon) into each cube. Freeze overnight. Place herb ice cubes in labeled freezer bags. These work well added to soups, stews or sauces.

Herbal Vinegars and Olive Oils

Simply place a small handful or a few sprigs of fresh (rinsed and dried) herbs into an 8-ounce jar of apple cider vinegar, white wine vinegar, white balsamic vinegar or extra virgin olive oil. Store in airtight jars, labeled for contents and date. Hardy herbs such as rosemary and thyme may stay in the jars. Remove leafy herbs such as basil and parsley after 1 to 2 weeks. No need to refrigerate. Use within 6 months.

Herb Butters

Experiment with different herb combinations and create butters from your favorites. Remove leaves from stems, keeping the stems for later use in a broth.

Chop herbs finely. Melt a stick of butter in a saucepan over medium heat. Sauté herbs gently over low heat for a few minutes, then remove from heat. Pour the melted butter and herbs into a large glass mixing bowl and whisk for one minute. Pour the mixture into labeled baby food jars. Stir while the jar is cooling. Refrigerate once the butter has cooled. If you desire whipped butter, simply whip the melted herb butter in a food processor and refrigerate in baby food jars.

Pesto

Pesto is a simple way to prolong the freshness of herbs. According to the *Etymology Dictionary,* pesto got its name from *pestato,* past participle of *pestare* "to pound, to crush" (from the Latin root of *pestle*), in reference to the crushed herbs and garlic ingredients. It can be made from basil, parsley, cilantro, chervil, dill, mint or lemon balm, as well as from lettuce, arugula, kale, chard or wild edible weeds such as lamb's quarters and chickweed.

BASIC PESTO

> 6 cups fresh herbs (leaves only)
> 1 cup nuts (pine nuts are standard, but use any nuts or sunflower
>   or pumpkin seeds)
> 1 cup extra virgin olive oil
> 2 cloves garlic
> Pinch of salt
> 1 tablespoon lemon juice, to preserve freshness

Combine ingredients in a food processor until desired consistency. Adjust to your personal taste and desired texture. Adding more oil and lemon juice, for instance, will make the pesto runnier. Using less will make a more spreadable pesto for sandwiches or bagels. Freeze excess pesto in labeled freezer bags or ice cube trays. Place the cubes in a labeled freezer bag. Thaw and use as needed.

Try the following recipes, inspired by herbalist Colleen Smith's lamb's quarters pesto.

(Previously published in *Mother Earth News*.)

WILD AND GOURMET GREENS PESTO

> 4 cups wild and gourmet greens (equal amounts of chickweed,
>   lamb's quarters, spinach and leaf lettuce)
> Pinch of Celtic sea salt
> 1 cup extra virgin olive oil
> ½ cup toasted nuts
> 6 cloves garlic, toasted

Blend the greens and salt in the food processor, then slowly add the remaining ingredients. Purée until the desired consistency is reached.

PEPPERMINT PESTO

> 4 cups peppermint leaves (any mint will do)
> ½ teaspoon organic sugar or honey
> 1 cup extra virgin olive oil

Blend the mint and sugar in the food processor, then slowly add the remaining ingredients. Purée until the desired consistency is reached. Peppermint pesto is excellent served on homemade brownies or natural vanilla ice cream.

If you have mint growing in your yard, take advantage of it! Peppermint has a cooling effect on the body, is great for the digestive system and helps to soothe fevers. It is also great with lemon balm in herb-infused water.

ARUGULA, LEMON AND ARTICHOKE PESTO

> 6 cups arugula
> ½ cup extra virgin olive oil
> ½ cup toasted nuts
> 6 cloves garlic, toasted
> 1 can of artichoke hearts packed in oil (don't throw out the oil)
> 1 lemon, juiced
> Pinch of Celtic sea salt

Blend the greens and salt in the food processor, then slowly add the remaining ingredients. Purée until the desired consistency is reached.

GARLIC SCAPE PESTO

> 10 garlic scapes
> 1 cup extra virgin olive oil
> Pinch of sea salt
> Handful of fresh herbs (basil and parsley work well)
> Handful of pine nuts (optional)
> ¼ cup Asiago or Parmesan cheese (optional)

Combine in the food processor or blender for 1 minute.

Use garlic scapes just as you would use garlic. Chop, dice, blend or roast, or cook them whole in soups and stews. Blend with olive oil, vinegar and fresh herbs for a tangy salad dressing!

More Pesto Ideas!

◉ Mix pesto with olive oil and vinegar for a delicious salad dressing.
◉ Mix pesto with a cream sauce for a delicious pesto Alfredo.
◉ Use pesto as a spread on sandwiches, bagels and wraps.
◉ Mix pesto with sun-dried tomatoes to make sun-dried tomato pesto.
◉ Add pesto to macaroni and cheese or lasagna.

Our kids love pesto and can eat it by the spoonful. After trying Colleen's delicious lamb's quarters pesto, I started throwing all kinds of greens into my pesto, such as spinach, chard, kale and even gourmet salad mix, to sneak those nutrient-packed greens into the kids' daily meals.

During the winter, when basil is not available by the armful, take any pesto recipe and replace it with spinach, kale, chard, kale, lettuce and even wild greens such as chickweed!

Preserving Food

Oftentimes I hear that individuals don't have time to cook. Cooking can become all-consuming, but it doesn't have to be. There is value in home-cooked meals!

Homegrown, home-cooked meals not only taste better than processed and packaged foods loaded with pesticides, preservatives and ingredients that are difficult to pronounce, but they are better for the environment. Choosing to cook with food you've grown or bought from a local farm significantly reduces the number of travel miles and resources needed. Growing your own food truly reduces your carbon footprint in a very significant way.

Below are some ways that you contribute positively to the environment through supporting local food:

- Reducing reliance on fossil fuels
- Localizing your food supply
- Supporting the local economy
- Reducing reliance on corporations
- Withdrawing support of pesticide and herbicide usage

Helpful Supplies for Putting Up Food for the Winter

Things to acquire by purchasing, combing Craigslist, bartering or finding at thrift stores:

- Wide-mouth Mason jars in all sizes
- Canning pot/canning basket/canning tongs
- Shelving for canned goods

Things best when bought new:

- Pressure canner
- Standard Mason jar lids and rings (for canning)
- Plastic Mason jar lids (for freezing, reusing jars and fermentation)
- Freezer-safe bags
- Reusable freezer-safe containers with lids

Resourcefulness from the Garden to the Kitchen

I have enjoyed challenging myself to create beautiful gourmet meals without feeling the dire urge to go to the grocery store, but instead just opening the pantry and the refrigerator to see what ingredients I already have on hand. This not only saves money, but it also frees up time to spend with my family.

For example, say the family is craving pasta. I open the pantry, and there is no pasta. I muster up the motivation and spend the gas money and the time to go to the grocery store and face the inevitable "went in for one thing, came out with a cartful" that we all have experienced. My alternative is to figure out a creative way to use what I have on hand, like making a similar dish with a whole grain instead of pasta. Or slicing vegetables such as zucchini, squash or even sweet potatoes to resemble pasta. It can be challenging but creatively rewarding.

Eating with the seasons requires dedication to the environment, commitment to your health and a newfound creativity in the kitchen. Trying new recipes is a classic way to conquer picky eating habits. A surefire way to get on board with the local foods movement is to broaden your horizons by changing the way you see your food. The seasonal produce that grows throughout the world at specific seasons should be revered as foodshed miracles.

Eat with the Seasons: Get Creative in the Kitchen

When discovering the newfound excitement of eating with the seasons, we have the opportunity to get a little more creative in our own kitchens. I make most of our meals primarily with the vegetables we grow ourselves, minus the occasional gourmet ingredients such as various cheeses and staples such as oils and vinegars. I used to carry around a mile-long grocery list with me. After living and working on a vegetable farm for so long, I have done without most items on that list. As it turns out, we are perfectly content with a primarily vegetarian diet prepared with farm-fresh seasonal veggies that are abundant, tasty and beautiful.

Create beautiful home-cooked gourmet meals from seed to table. Create amazing new recipes by pairing the foods in your bountiful harvest. Create your own value-added products such as pestos, jams, jellies, preserves, sauces, salsas and so much more.

Tips on Preserving Autumn's Garden Bounty

The autumn equinox sends a signal to the backyard gardener's cerebral cortex, gently reminding us that the harvest season has arrived and that now is the time to be preserving and putting up food for the winter. Within just a couple of short months, the garden will once again become dormant and barren, giving the soil a time to rest. An avid gardener's greatest bounty occurs at this time of year. The seasoned homesteaders and canners have it down to a science, putting up multiple jars of tomatoes, sauces, salsas, fruits, vegetables, jams and jellies. Hats off to those folks. Becoming skilled in this age-old hobby requires knowledge of safety measures and temperature regulation to prevent risks of botulism and temperamental pressure canners.

For beginners, it is best to stick to hot water-bath canning, an age-old art passed down from generation to generation. I was taught by my homesteading hero friend, Colleen Smith, who lives with her husband and their three beautiful daughters in the two-room schoolhouse her grandparents both attended decades ago. Colleen is a master herbalist and avid gardener who has been canning tomatoes since she was a teenager. Her father is the king of tomatoes, winning many blue ribbons for best tomatoes. Colleen uses a portable propane cooker or turkey fryer to can like a rock star.

When canning at home, it is best to take a class in your community first. There are many important things to know such as sterilization techniques, proper temperatures, safety methods and just good general tips.

Canned Vegetables

(makes 3 to 6 quarts)

Place a large canning pot on a propane cooker or on your stovetop. Place a canning rack inside the pot and add 6 to 8 jars. Fill pot with water about ¾ full, making sure the jars are fully submerged to sterilize them. Turn heat on to medium high. Bring water to a boil. Use canning tongs to remove jars and lay them right side up on a towel to air dry.

Sterilize lids and rings in a separate small saucepan of boiling water.

Fill a separate large stainless steel pot with boiling water. Add 6 quarts of vegetables.

Boil vegetables for about 3–5 minutes and strain.

Re-boil the pot used to sterilize jars (you will use this to can tomatoes).

Fill sterilized jars with vegetables. Leave about ½ inch breathing room at the top.

Using a clean cloth, dip an end into boiled water to wipe the rims before adding the lids. Once they are securely fastened, arrange jars of vegetables on the canning rack. Carefully place it into the large pot of boiling water and process for about 45 minutes.

Using canning tongs, remove jars from the hot water bath. Place them on a towel to dry.

Be sure that the lid sinks inward in a concave direction. Listen for the popping sound that occurs once the jar has sealed. If you can push the lid down like a button, it has not sealed. Jars need to be sealed completely. If you have trouble getting them to seal all the way, you can always pour the contents into a freezer-safe Ziploc bag and freeze them. Don't forget to label your jars and your freezer bags with the contents and the date.

For more homesteading ideas and tips on canning, preserving and foraging wild edibles, visit Colleen and Jamie's blog at Wildstead.wordpress.com.

Freezing

Freezing is an underutilized and excellent way to preserve your garden bounty — and it's virtually foolproof. For squash, potatoes, sweet potatoes or eggplant, fully cook or blanch them and freeze in a freezer bag for quick meal additions. For peppers, corn or onions, just chop and freeze them to later add to omelettes, quiches, stir-fries or other meals. This will make meal preparation more convenient, too!

With your harvest, cook large batches of soups or stews and freeze in freezer bags to thaw and heat in any amount you desire. Try new seasonal recipes such as hearty autumn stew, sweet potato pancakes, roasted butternut squash with lemon butter sauce, roasted butternut squash bisque topped with pan-fried sage, sweet apple and wild rice-stuffed acorn squash, and any other fall-inspired dishes that you have been eager to make.

Autumn Stew

1 gallon of water
¼ cup hard cider or white wine
Salt and pepper to taste
Pinch of pumpkin pie spice
Pinch of ground cloves
Pinch of cumin (optional)
3 large sweet potatoes, sliced or cubed
3 large tomatoes, cut in half and sliced
4 medium peppers, sliced

Boil water, cider and seasonings in a large saucepan. Add sweet potatoes. Cook for 10 minutes over medium heat. Add remaining ingredients and cook on low for 45 minutes.

Grilling

We love the flavor of campfire veggies. It is a great way to use up any with blemishes. A simple way to build your own campstove is with cinder blocks, stone or firebricks stacked in a ring about a foot high. Be sure you build it so your grill can rest securely on top. For example, if your grill top is 24 inches in diameter, build a ring with fire bricks that is 23 inches in diameter. If you're not worried about the "campfire flavor," simply BBQ the veggies. Eat them immediately or chop and freeze them to add to hearty soups, stews, chili or pasta. Oak, cedar and cherry woods all have great flavor and are Farmer Eric's favorite!

(Excerpts from below were originally published in *Feast Magazine*.)

There is nothing more nostalgic than the smell of a campfire. The aroma of oak, hickory, cherry and cedar burning while the smoke rises; the glow of the embers that tells you it's time to start grilling; the scent that lingers on your clothes for days. The campfire smell brings back so many fond childhood memories of camping in the Missouri Ozarks, wading in the creek all day and cooking on cast-iron skillets at dusk, stars shining brightly, listening to the symphony orchestra of wildlife through the night.

Compared to charcoal grilling, cooking with wood may just be a lost art, but the robust flavors attained by wood-fired grilling are enhanced tenfold.

Eric and I tend to use reclaimed and repurposed materials in each of our creative endeavors. We built a multi-functioning firepit/outdoor wood-fired barbeque grill using large found stones and a circular grill from an old BBQ pit. We use our wood-fired grill regularly throughout spring, summer and fall. That fire-roasted flavor enhances any dish. One of the many perks of being farmers is that we get to intercept a plethora of slightly blemished veggies from going to the compost pile. We simply cut off the blemished parts, toss the rest in olive oil and a little sea salt and throw them on the grill.

Wood-fired veggies are a great way to use seasonal bounty and make an excellent addition to soups, stews, pasta salads and sides. Preserve them by freezing in freezer-safe bags.

Peppers are among our favorite vegetables to grill during the late summer months, when they are at their peak flavor and ripeness. We use these three methods:

- Fire-roasted on the wood-fired grill (4 minutes on each side)
- Fire-roasted on the charcoal grill (4 minutes on each side)
- Roasted in the oven (toss in extra virgin olive oil and a pinch of salt and bake at 425°F for 20 minutes)

We prefer to use jalapeño, poblano and Anaheim peppers. It is best to leave them whole, toss them in olive oil and sea salt, and grill on each side for about 4 minutes, until they have slightly flattened, are tender and have nice charred grill marks. Remove from grill and let cool for at least 30 minutes. Cut off the stems and remove seeds. Rinse slightly.

Fire-roasted Hot Pepper Paste

24 fire-roasted jalapeños (preferably red)
6 fire-roasted poblano peppers
2 tablespoons red wine vinegar
1 teaspoon Celtic sea salt

In a food processor, combine all ingredients and process for 1 minute or until smooth and creamy. The paste will stay good refrigerated in a tightly sealed jar for up to 2 weeks. It freezes well in freezer-safe bags.

Spicy Chow Chow with Fire-roasted Hot Peppers

2 large onions, diced
4 cloves of garlic, minced
¼ cup extra virgin olive oil
1 green cabbage, cut in half lengthwise and grilled
3 small summer squash, cut in half lengthwise and grilled
3 fire-roasted poblano peppers, diced
5 fire-roasted jalapeño peppers, diced
2 fire-roasted bell peppers, diced
1 tablespoon Celtic sea salt
1 teaspoon cracked black pepper
1 tablespoon sugar (I prefer coconut sugar)

In a large pot, sauté onions and garlic in oil for 2 minutes. Chop grilled cabbage and squash and add to the pot. Cook on medium heat for 2 minutes. Add diced fire-roasted hot and bell peppers, salt, pepper and sugar. Cook on medium heat for 5 minutes or until all ingredients are tender. Chow chow will keep refrigerated for 1 week in a tightly sealed jar. It freezes well in freezer-safe bags.

Don't forget about your freezer. Make batches of sauces or salsas and freeze in labeled freezer bags. Grill a large quantity of veggies, cut into strips and freeze in labeled freezer bags to have the taste of summer any time of the year.

GOURMET PASTA SAUCE

(makes 6 batches)

> 4 onions, chopped
> 24 cloves of garlic, minced
> 15–20 peppers, chopped
> ¼ cup extra virgin olive oil
> ¼ cup red wine
> ¼ cup red wine vinegar
> 1 small bunch of each fresh herb: parsley, oregano, thyme, basil
>   and sage, chopped
> 4 tablespoons Celtic sea salt
> ½ cup brown sugar or coconut sugar
> 70–100 tomatoes (peeled using the hot water method) OR
> 3–5 gallons of Sungold cherry tomatoes (no need to peel)

Sauté onions, garlic and peppers in olive oil. Add wine and vinegar and simmer for 5 minutes. Add chopped fresh herbs, salt and sugar and simmer for 5 minutes. Add this mixture to tomatoes in a large stock pot. Bring to a boil. Cook on medium heat for about 25 minutes or until everything is tender. Simmer for 10 minutes on low heat. Let mixture cool to room temperature. You may process this mixture in the blender to achieve the desired consistency. Separate into Ziploc bags, label the contents and dates.

For the Love of Fermentation

Lacto-fermentation is the process of fermenting veggies in lactic acid-forming bacteria that are beneficial to the body and help build the immune system.

PRESERVED VEGGIES IN BRINE

> Sterilize Mason jars.
> Chop veggies and herbs of your choice and add to jars.
> Dissolve 1½ tablespoons of Celtic sea salt in 2 cups of purified
>   water.
> Pour the brine over your chopped veggies in the jars.
> Leave ½ inch of space at the top. Put a cabbage leaf on top to
>   help with the fermentation process.
> Cover with a plastic lid.
> Leave on the counter for 1 week.
> Remove cabbage leaf and refrigerate for up to 2 months. Be sure
>   to label.

SAUERKRAUT IN MASON JARS

(Adapted from recipe by Emma Christensen of Kitchn) (thekitchen.com)

> 3 large heads green cabbage
> 4 tablespoons sea salt or kosher salt
> 1 tablespoon freshly cracked black pepper
> 4 tablespoons caraway seeds
> 2 dried cayenne peppers, seeds removed and cut into strips with
>   Scissors (optional)

Have the following on hand before you begin:

> Large cutting board
> Large sharp knife (I find a nice large serrated knife works best for
>   cutting thin strips of cabbage)
> giant mixing bowl
> Measuring spoons/measuring cup
> Canning funnel
> 6 large sterilized one-quart wide-mouth Mason jars and plastic
>   lids
> Muslin or butter muslin cheesecloth
> 6 large rubber bands
> 6 sterilized jelly jars that can fit into a wide-mouth Mason jar
> 1 bag of marbles (used to keep the cabbage beneath its own
>   juices)

Wash everything you will be using very well. Sterilize jars. Cut the ends off the heads of cabbage. Slice very thin and place in the large bowl. Add the salt evenly over it and mix by hand for at least 8 minutes. The desired result is slightly wilted and juicy cabbage in a fair amount of liquid.

Put the cabbage into the Mason jars using the canning funnel, about ¾ full. Evenly pour the remaining liquid from the mixing bowl into each jar. Place a folded cabbage leaf over the surface of the shredded cabbage. It should be completely immersed in its own liquid.

Divide the marbles equally between the six jelly jars. Place them inside each of the jars with cabbage. Use a wooden spoon to press the jelly jar down firmly, watching the liquid level rise.

Cut muslin or cheesecloth into 6 squares (4x4 inches), cover the jars and secure with a rubber band.

Over the next few days, every couple of hours, or whenever you remember, press the smaller jar firmly down, allowing the juices to rise above the cabbage.

If the liquid levels are not above the cabbage after two days, mix 1 tablespoon of salt with 1 cup of distilled water and pour it into each Mason jar, making sure the liquid covers the cabbage.

Ferment the cabbage for 7–12 days, keeping it out of direct sunlight and at a temperature that is between 60° and 75°F.

Check to make sure the liquid level stays above the cabbage. This is very important for fermentation and preventing slime mold. Once fermentation has occurred to your desired taste, remove smaller jars of marbles and the large folded leaves. Transfer the sauerkraut to smaller containers and add the plastic caps. Refrigerate and enjoy. Use within 4–6 months.

Integrating Probiotics into Your Kids' Diet

(Adapted from the Domestic Diva blog)

- Add kefir grains to juice (kefir grains eat the sugar and leave behind bubbles).
- Make homemade ketchup using tomatoes and dates. Add probiotics to it and let it sit on the counter for two days. Probiotics from whey eat all of the sugar.
- Let them help you make lacto-fermented vegetables.
- Allow them to choose their favorite vegetables to add to the jars.
- Use organic sourdough bread.
- Try raw organic cheese and probiotic pickles.
- Add kefir to smoothies.
- Use cultured fruits and fruit leathers, carrots and applesauce.
- Try kombucha in small amounts.
- Add probiotic supplements.
- Make homemade probiotic yogurt.

Raw Power Foods

Incorporating plenty of raw fresh organically grown fruits and vegetables into your diet is essential for optimal health! They are loaded with vital nutrients; packed full of vitamins and minerals; contain chlorophyll, probiotics, digestive enzymes and antioxidants; and are an excellent source of fiber.

Permaculture in the Kitchen

My favorite example of retraining yourself to eat with the seasons is zucchini noodles. When zucchini is in season, I don't even keep pasta stocked in the pantry because zucchini noodles are delicious and healthy; my entire family loves them and asks for seconds. Getting kids to eat healthy can be a challenge, but it is always a little easier when they can be involved in the process. I love preparing raw food meals using farm-fresh produce during the summer to be sure we get the maximum nutrients and flavor. One of my favorite ways is to make a raw version of fettuccini Alfredo using thinly sliced zucchini as the noodles, topped with a cashew and basil cream sauce.

Zucchini squash can be served hot or cold, raw or cooked, shredded, sliced, cubed or diced. It can be baked, broiled, fried, sautéed, steamed and grilled. As if the zucchini weren't impressive enough, even the blossom is edible. In addition to its beauty and flavor, zucchini is a highly nutritious vegetable with excellent antioxidant properties as well, containing generous amounts of vitamins A, C and B-complex, as well as iron, manganese and zinc.

Zucchini Noodles

Use a spiral slicer or score large zucchini lengthwise with a paring knife all the way. Use a handheld vegetable peeler to slice "noodles" from top to bottom. Use them in place of noodles in any recipe. You can serve them hot or cold, with pesto or the sauce of your choice. My three favorites are pesto, a cashew-based Alfredo sauce and a raw sun-dried tomato and date sauce.

Cashew Alfredo Sauce

> 2 cups raw cashews
> Pinch of Celtic sea salt
> ½ lemon, juiced
> 2 cups purified water

In a food processor, blend cashews until finely crumbled. Slowly add salt, fresh lemon juice and water until the mixture is smooth and creamy. Add a splash more water if necessary to achieve creaminess.

Pesto Cream Sauce

Make cashew Alfredo sauce from recipe above. Add 6 tablespoons of pesto and blend until smooth.

SUN-DRIED TOMATO AND DATE SAUCE

 1 cup sun-dried tomatoes
 ¼ cup pitted dried dates
 3 cloves garlic
 Pinch of Celtic sea salt
 1 cup purified water

In a food processor, blend sun-dried tomatoes and dates until they are roughly chopped. Add garlic, salt and water and blend until the mixture resembles pasta sauce.

Chard can be a substitute for a tortilla or bread and tastes great with any savory filling. I like to serve omelettes on a chard roll and let the whole family roll their own breakfast burritos. Chard is beautifully matched with lemony flavors and neutralized by cream cheeses or soft cheeses such as goat chèvre or brie. It can also be sautéed with onions and garlic, chopped and added to soups, or chopped and served in a salad. Collards, kale or cabbage leaves may also be used.

CHARD ROLLS WITH NUTTY RANCH DIPPING SAUCE

 12 large chard leaves
 2 cups fresh greens of your choice
 1 cup local mushrooms
 2 cloves garlic, minced
 ½ cup sliced colorful peppers
 ½ cup sprouts or micro greens
 ½ cup chopped vegetables of your choice

Rinse and dry chard leaves.

Cut the tip of the stem adjoining the leaf in an upside down V shape (you don't want the stem in your rolls because it might rip the leaf, causing the wrap to fall apart.) Lay the chard leaves (shiny side down) next to one another on a large flat surface.

Combine remaining ingredients in a large mixing bowl. Place 4 large spoonfuls of the mixture onto each leaf (toward the end where you cut a V shape).

Roll up like a burrito and use a toothpick to hold each one in place.

Nutty Ranch Dipping Sauce

1 cup raw cashews
¼ cup purified water
2 tablespoons dried or fresh herbs of your choice (I use a mixture
of fresh dill, parsley, thyme, oregano and cilantro)
Pinch of Celtic sea salt

In a food processor, blend the cashews until they are finely crumbled. Slowly add the remaining ingredients. Add a splash more water if necessary to make the mixture smooth and creamy but not too thin.

Raw Power Slaw

A great way to use your farm veggies is to make a delicious raw slaw. You can flavor it any way you'd like.

I start with thinly sliced or shaved veggies, oil, vinegar, sea salt and cracked pepper. I like to make a variety of slaws: curry raisin, Asian sesame, fresh herb and apple cider vinegar, etc.... Get creative! Be resourceful and challenge yourself to use what you have in your kitchen!

Vegan Caesar Salad

4 handfuls spring greens, washed and spun
1 avocado, finely chopped
2 garlic cloves, minced
5 tablespoons vegan mayo
Pinch of Celtic sea salt
Dash of freshly ground black pepper

Toss all ingredients together and top with handmade croutons and hemp seeds.

Spring Detox Salad

(For best results, use all organic ingredients)

4 handfuls spring greens, washed and spun
1 handful raw pumpkin seeds
¼ cup shredded red cabbage
¼ cup chopped raw cauliflower
1 avocado, chopped

Toss all ingredients together and serve with Spring Detox Dressing.

SPRING DETOX DRESSING

> ¼ cup apple cider vinegar
>
> ¼ cup flax oil
>
> 2 tablespoons dill weed
>
> 1 tablespoon raw honey
>
> 1 lemon, juiced

Mix all ingredients together.

SPICY KALE CHIPS

> 2 cups raw cashews
>
> 1 cup raw sunflower seeds
>
> ¾ cup raw sesame seeds
>
> ½ cup sun-dried tomatoes
>
> 6 figs
>
> ¼ cup raw pumpkin seeds

Soak above ingredients in distilled water for about an hour.

> 6 cloves garlic
>
> 2 stalks celery
>
> 2 carrots
>
> ½ cup melted coconut oil or avocado oil
>
> 4 tablespoons Bragg's apple cider vinegar
>
> 4 tablespoons Bragg's liquid aminos
>
> 1 tablespoon ground red pepper
>
> 1 lemon, juiced
>
> 2 cups nutritional yeast
>
> 2 tablespoons poppy seeds
>
> Water as needed
>
> 6 heads curly kale

Blend soaked ingredients (including the water) as well as garlic, celery and carrot in a food processor until smooth. Add remaining ingredients, except kale. Add extra water if you need to. The mixture should be a thick paste.

Remove stems and tear kale into large pieces. Wash well and dry with a large towel. In a large bowl, combine with the paste.

Place the coated kale on food dehydrator layers. Dehydrate for at least six hours. The kale chips should be crispy.

Bake any extra coated kale on the lowest setting in an oven for an hour or until crispy.

SUSHI

Sushi is a great way to eat your veggies. Simply cut peppers, squash, cucumbers, green beans and any other veggie you wish into matchsticks.

Cook sushi rice according to package instructions. (Make it raw by substituting rice with cauliflower pulsed in the food processor — add a handful of cashews to make the mixture sticky.)

Place nori sheet onto dry cutting board. Spread sushi rice evenly onto it with a spatula. Add veggies. Roll sushi using a bamboo sushi roller or simply use a large Ziploc bag. Cut with a sharp knife.

Raw Desserts

RAW CHOCOLATE FUDGE

2 cups coconut oil (melted)
1 cup raw cacao powder
4 tablespoons raw honey or pure maple syrup

In a mixing bowl, combine the coconut oil, raw cacao and honey or maple syrup until smooth. Pour into a freezer-safe glass dish and freeze for at least an hour. Serve immediately. Keep refrigerated.

RAW FOODS PIE CRUST

2 cups almonds
1 cup pitted dates, chopped
3 tablespoons pure maple syrup

In a food processor, blend almonds on high until they resemble flour. Add dates and maple syrup and blend until it forms a sticky ball. Grease a pie pan with coconut oil. Press the mixture into the pie pan to form a crust.

RAW CHOCOLATE MOUSSE

4 avocados
4 tablespoons cacao powder
3 tablespoons pure maple syrup

Blend in a blender or a food processor until smooth and creamy.

MULBERRY CASHEW CRÈME CHEESECAKE

(originally published in *Feast Magazine*)

Crust:

2 cups raw almonds

1½ cups dried mission figs, stems removed and then chopped

1 cup almond flour

1 teaspoon coconut oil

In a food processor, blend almonds on high until they resemble flour. Add chopped dried figs and almond flour and blend until the mixture has formed a sticky ball.

Use about a teaspoon of coconut oil to grease a glass pie dish. Press the crust mixture firmly down until it is evenly spread over the pie pan to form a crust.

Filling:

5 cups raw cashews

1 lemon, juiced

12 tablespoons honey or pure maple syrup (set 2 tablespoons
    aside to drizzle over the finished cheesecake)

3 tablespoons pure vanilla extract

1½ cups coconut milk or water

3 cups mulberries

1 tablespoon coconut oil

In a food processor, blend the cashews until they resemble a fine powder. Add the remaining filling ingredients (except mulberries and coconut oil) and blend on high until smooth and creamy. Set aside half of the filling in a small bowl. Add 2 cups of mulberries to the remaining filling mixture and continue to blend on high until creamy and colorful.

Pour the mulberry-tinted filling over the crust and spread evenly, saving about ½ cup for topping.

Spread the cashew crème filling evenly over the colored filling. Add the remaining ½ cup of mulberry-tinted filling on top in the center. Using a toothpick, slowly move it from center to edge using a swirling motion. Be creative. There is no right or wrong way to do this. Drizzle the cheesecake with honey or maple syrup.

Finally, arrange the remaining mulberries on top. I like to line them around the outside edge with a few in the center. Cover and refrigerate for at least an hour. Serve chilled.

My friends Chris Meyer and Mike Miller at Kitchen Kulture in St. Louis, MO started a business to bridge the gap between farmer and consumer. They create fresh delicious ready to go meals and sides using locally sourced ingredients. They are a perfect example of how eating with the seasons can be flavorful, quick and delicious. Their food is among the most unforgettable dining experiences I've ever had. Luckily, their booth is across from ours at the Tower Grove Farmers Market so we are fueled by their samples of fermented foods and global inspired farm-to-table cuisine. They have seasonal eating down to a science. Their menu changes with the seasons and they are continuously coming up with new ways to use produce and meats directly from the farmer. They just opened a brick and mortar location called Kounter Kulture. Check them out at www.Kitchenkulturestl.com

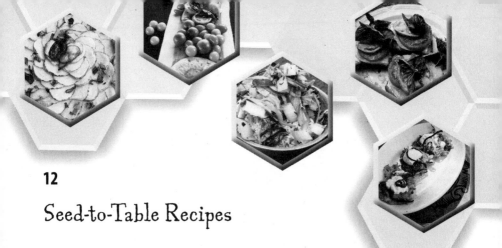

12

Seed-to-Table Recipes

Breakfast Dishes

SWEET POTATO PANCAKES

Peel, boil and mash 3 medium sweet potatoes. Add them to your favorite pancake recipe (decreasing wet ingredients by ¼). They turn out best when cooked in butter on a cast-iron griddle.

CHARD AND KALE OMELETTE

Chard and kale are so versatile; chop them up and throw them into any savory dish. One of my favorites is to cut leaves fine with scissors and whisk with 4 or 5 eggs, a splash of cream, goat cheese, minced garlic, roasted red peppers and baby Swiss chard. Our kids clear their plates every time!

Use chard and kale like spinach, fresh or raw! Finely cut and add to stir-fries, soups, salads, pesto, pastas, spanakopita and artichoke dip.

SUMMER BREAKFAST HASH

Sauté finely chopped potatoes, sweet potatoes and onions in olive oil for 15 minutes. Add finely chopped squash and peppers. Sauté for 10 minutes. Top with a diced tomato, fresh basil and parsley. Add a farm egg for extra protein. Optional: garnish with shredded cheese, hot sauce and a dollop of vegan mayo.

Seasonal Veggie Egg Bake

Farm-fresh eggs are the most amazing we have ever had. Egg bakes can be made quickly the night before using dinner leftovers.

> 1 dozen farm eggs
> ¼ cup cream or milk (or substitute)
> 1 cup of bread cubes (could be day old bread)
> Roasted veggies (leftovers from dinner)
> Handful of hardy greens, such as spinach, kale or chard
> ½ cup cheese (cut into small pieces)
> Pinch of salt (optional)
> Herbs (optional)

Grease a baking dish and preheat the oven to 400°F.

Whisk together eggs and cream. Add remaining ingredients and stir well. Pour mixture into baking dish and cook for 25–30 minutes or until the eggs have set in the middle.

You can also make the mixture the night before but stir in bread cubes and refrigerate in a covered baking dish.

Snacks

Farmer Eric's Famous Radish Dip

Farmer Eric loves radishes… especially when minced and mixed with cream cheese! We grow the bright pink ones called red meat or watermelon radishes at La Vista.

> 1 8-ounce package goat cheese, softened
> 6 radishes, minced
> 2 scallions, sliced thin
> 1 small bunch of chives
> 2 teaspoons poppyseeds
> Pinch of salt

Combine all ingredients and serve on crackers, Melba toast or with cucumber tea sandwiches.

Vegetarian Buffalo Chicken Dip

> 4 cups sautéed squash and onions
> 1 cup shredded cheddar cheese
> ¼ cup Buffalo-style hot sauce (such as Frank's)

Combine all ingredients in a baking dish and cook for 20 minutes at 425°F.

VEGAN SWEET POTATO PUB CHEESE

(originally published in *Feast Magazine*)

Sweet potatoes are a very versatile vegetable. They can be sliced with a spiral slicer to make noodles and are actually amazing when eaten raw with the right spices. Cook them whole, roasted, baked, boiled, fried, sautéed, steamed and shredded.

Chips and rarebit are one of my weaknesses, but only in moderation since they aren't exactly a health food. Luckily, boiled sweet potatoes when blended with a few ingredients can taste so much like a pub cheese or rarebit, you may forget it's a healthy alternative. Served with baked Yukon gold potato rounds, they make a perfect pair when starch is what you crave.

> 6 medium-large sweet potatoes, peeled
> 1 cup hemp milk or other milk/milk substitute
> 1 tablespoon sea salt
> 1 teaspoon black pepper
> 1 tablespoon smoked paprika
> ½ cup dark beer
> 1 teaspoon Bragg's liquid aminos or tamari soy sauce (for a richer flavor)

Cut sweet potatoes into 1-inch cubes and boil until slightly soft (about 25 minutes).

Drain, keeping the broth to add later or as a broth for other recipes.

Place potatoes and remaining ingredients (except the beer) into a food processor. Pulse until smooth. Process on high for 2 minutes, adding a little more of the sweet potato water to thin if necessary.

In a medium saucepan on low, slowly add the beer to the sweet potato "cheese," stirring regularly for about 5 minutes.

While the sweet potatoes boil, create your chips.

BAKED YUKON GOLD POTATO ROUNDS

> 6 Yukon gold potatoes
> 1 teaspoon sea salt
> Extra virgin olive oil
> Fresh sage, pan-fried (optional)

Preheat oven to 425°F. Wash the potatoes and cut into ¼-inch slices. Toss in a large bowl with sea salt and enough olive oil to evenly coat them. Place them in a single layer on a baking sheet. Bake for about 25 minutes or until tender and slightly crispy on the edges. Broil for 1–2 minutes until golden and a little crisper. Top with pan-fried sage.

Hearty Salads: Nutritious. Delicious. Hundreds of Ways to Prepare!

(The following two recipes originally published in *Feast Magazine*)

Fruits and Blooms

Nothing says welcome to summer like fresh-picked strawberries! Add strawberries to a refreshing spinach salad with sliced crisp apples, dandelion flowers, candied or raw walnuts and cashews, and maple fig balsamic dressing! Our kids can never get enough "Strawberry Fields Forever"!

Beautiful brunch salads are a scrumptious way to devour the delicate blossoms of spring alongside the fruits of a farmer's labor. Fresh, gourmet mixed greens, which are available locally in the summer, provide a neutral base for a flavorful salad topped with sweet and sophisticated fruit, blossoms, nuts and cheeses.

STRAWBERRY DANDELION BRUNCH SALAD WITH MAPLE FIG BALSAMIC DRESSING

> 1 pound fresh salad greens, washed and spun (organic are best)
> 15 medium ripe strawberries, sliced lengthways (organic are best)
> 10–15 fresh-picked dandelion flowers, washed and dried
> ½ cup shelled pecan halves (candied optional)
> 3 ounces fresh goat chèvre, separated with a knife into small pieces (or crumbled goat or feta cheese)

This salad is best served on a large shallow platter to showcase its beauty. Arrange the greens evenly on your platter. Layer the pecans, strawberries and goat cheese and top with the maple fig dressing. Garnish with the dandelion flowers.

CREAMY MAPLE FIG BALSAMIC DRESSING

> 1 cup extra virgin olive oil
> ¾ cup balsamic vinegar
> ¼ cup pure maple syrup (local syrup is frequently available at
>   farmers' markets)
> 12 dried figs, hard tips removed

In a blender, combine all ingredients, processing one minute or until completely smooth and creamy. Add more olive oil and blend again if necessary. Taste the mixture to assure desired flavor is achieved, equal parts sweet and slightly sour, and adjust recipe accordingly. Refrigerate any extra in a Mason jar with a tight-fitting lid for up to three weeks.

SPINACH AND STRAWBERRY SALAD WITH EDIBLE FLOWERS

Add spinach to your salad greens and top with sliced strawberries, pecans and edible flowers such as nasturtiums. Serve with strawberry poppyseed dressing or balsamic vinaigrette.

STRAWBERRY POPPYSEED VINAIGRETTE

> 1 cup fresh strawberries, tops removed, washed and cut in half
> 1 cup extra virgin olive oil
> ½ cup white balsamic vinegar
> 2 tablespoons honey or maple syrup
> 6 tablespoons poppyseeds

In a blender or food processor, blend strawberries until they are smashed. Slowly add oil, vinegar and honey or maple syrup. Blend until smooth and creamy. Add poppyseeds and blend again. Refrigerate in Mason jars for up to a week or freeze. If freezing, thaw and blend again before serving.

ARTICHOKE AND ARUGULA SALAD WITH LEMON WHITE BALSAMIC VINAIGRETTE

Top a spicy salad blend with marinated artichoke hearts, farm-fresh scallions and chives (cut thin with scissors), sliced cucumbers, radishes and chive flowers.

LEMON WHITE BALSAMIC VINAIGRETTE

>   1 cup extra virgin olive oil
>   ½ cup white balsamic vinegar
>   Pinch of sea salt and pepper
>   1 teaspoon dill
>   1 teaspoon mustard seed
>   1 lemon, juiced

Whisk ingredients together in a bowl. Enjoy!

GRILLED RADICCHIO AND NAPA CABBAGE SALAD

Cut radicchio and cabbage in half. Brush with olive oil. Grill for a few minutes on each side. Cut into thin strips and toss in olive oil, apple cider vinegar, a pinch of salt, a pinch of pepper and a pinch of sugar. Add sriracha if you like a little spice.

RADISH, APPLE AND WALNUT SALAD WITH
OATMEAL STOUT HONEY BALSAMIC VINAIGRETTE

Salad in a jar: a simple on-the-go meal!

   Pour salad dressing into a Mason jar. Layer greens, red cabbage, carrots, sunflower seeds and whatever else you wish. Squeeze fresh lemon over greens to preserve freshness. Shake before eating.

GOLDEN ZUCCHINI, CUCUMBER AND BASIL SALAD

>   2 medium zucchini, cut into matchsticks
>   2 medium cucumber, cut into matchsticks
>   24 fresh basil leaves
>   1 cup cherry tomatoes, cut in half
>   ¼ cup white balsamic vinegar
>   ¼ cup extra virgin olive oil
>   Pinch of sea salt
>   Pinch of fresh cracked black pepper

Combine all ingredients in a bowl and serve with fried green tomatoes or baked and breaded zucchini.

Slaws

Zucchini and Carrot Slaw

½ green cabbage
1 medium zucchini
3 carrots
¼ cup apple cider vinegar
2 tablespoons olive oil
½ tablespoon honey
1 teaspoon cumin
Pinch of salt
½ bunch of scallions, chopped
Handful of chopped almonds

Shred vegetables and toss with remaining ingredients in a bowl.

Farmer's Favorite Cucumber and Cilantro Salsa

1 jalapeño pepper
1 cucumber
1 tomato
12 cherry tomatoes
Small bunch of cilantro (stems removed)
½ red onion
½ lime, juiced
Salt
Pinch of smoked paprika (optional)

Finely chop vegetables. Add seasonings. Toss with a splash of olive oil. This recipe is delightful!

FARMER'S FAVORITE FIRE-ROASTED HOT PEPPER AND TOMATILLO SALSA

36 fire-roasted tomatillos
6 fire-roasted jalapeño peppers
3 fire-roasted poblano peppers
1 fresh lime, squeezed
1 bunch fresh cilantro
1 teaspoon red wine vinegar
1 teaspoon Celtic sea salt
1 teaspoon sugar (I prefer coconut sugar)
1 teaspoon cracked black pepper
2 small red onions, diced
4 garlic cloves, minced

Blend everything except for the onions and garlic in a food processor on high for 1 minute or until thoroughly processed. Pour mixture into a large bowl. Add chopped onions and minced garlic. This salsa will keep refrigerated for roughly 1 week in a tightly sealed jar. It also freezes well in freezer-safe bags.

Soups

DAD'S DELICIOUS VEGETABLE SOUP

My father made the most amazing vegetable soup. I've tried many times and have come close but not once mastered his recipe, which was never written down. Here is my attempt.

10 cups water or broth
4 potatoes, cut into small cubes
4 carrots, sliced
1 onion, diced
4 stalks of celery, diced
1 pound fresh green beans, cut into thirds
3 beets, cubed
Greens from 3 beets, chopped
6 garlic cloves, minced
4 tomatoes, chopped

Bring water or broth to a boil. Add potatoes, carrots and onion. Cook for 10 minutes on medium heat. Add the remaining ingredients and simmer for 2 hours or until veggies are tender.

Potato, Leek and Artichoke Soup

World-class chefs go crazy over bunching leeks, which grow in a clump like scallions, because of their delicate texture and elegant allium flavor. We grow them because we have not had success with large leeks. Use them just as you would leeks or onions. I like to cut them into thin slices, using sharp kitchen scissors, to use raw in salads and receive their wonderful nutrients. They are rich in iron and vitamins K, A and C and an abundance of other nutrients.

I balance our healthy eating habits with a little gourmet foodie fun: I also like to flash-fry them in olive oil to garnish soups, pastas and pizzas.

> 16 potatoes, washed and sliced thin
> 1 large leek or 6 bunching leeks
> 2 tablespoons extra virgin olive oil
> 1 large onion, sliced thin
> 6 garlic cloves, sliced thin
> 6 cups vegetable broth
> 2 jars marinated artichokes
> 1 cup roasted red peppers
> 2 tablespoons smoked paprika
> 2 tablespoons sea salt
> 2 tablespoons cracked black pepper
> 6 tablespoons fresh or dried herbs (I like to use a combination of
>   dill, oregano and parsley)

Boil potatoes in a large pot of water for 15 minutes or until tender. Cut leeks with scissors and dip in cold water to remove silt. In a large skillet, sauté leeks in a splash of oil for 5 minutes. Add onions and garlic and sauté for another 5–10 minutes or until tender. Fill a large pot with 6 cups of vegetable broth or water. Add the remaining ingredients and simmer on low for 10–15 minutes or until the flavors have married.

Stuffed Squash Blossoms

(Previously published in *Feast Magazine*.)

Squash blossoms are not only beautiful and vibrant, but they are also edible, nutrient-rich and delicious! They are high in iron, calcium and vitamins A and C.

A timeless way to use squash blossoms is to stuff them with goat chèvre and lightly fry them in a drizzle of olive oil in a cast-iron skillet. The zephyr squash is one of my top five all-time favorite vegetables! Its painted elegant appearance is striking … one of nature's masterpieces.

Zucchini squash blossoms are regarded as a delicacy by chefs for their stunning appearance, unique flavor and incomparable texture. The blossom melts in your mouth, leaving undertones of sweet nuttiness. Zucchini, also known as courgettes, are gorgeous when prepared with the flower still intact. The most dramatic appearance can be achieved by using baby zucchini (less than three inches long) with blossoms attached. Lightly sauté them in olive oil. Their natural beauty speaks for itself plated next to any main dish.

The squash blossoms of both zucchini and summer squash are edible; however, zucchini blossoms are preferred because they are a little stouter and they last longer. The blossoms are highly perishable and should be prepared within a few hours of harvest. It is best to cut about ¼ inch of zucchini end with the blossom so that it remains intact and easy to use. They have such a unique and delightful flavor that they are best prepared with just one or two simple ingredients. They are excellent stuffed with any cheese, but my favorite is the simple delicate flavor of goat chèvre.

> 12 freshly harvested squash blossoms (optional: include the
>   3–5 inch zucchini)
> 1 4-ounce package goat chèvre
> 4 tablespoons extra virgin olive oil

Preheat the oven to 350°F. Coat a sheet pan with a thin layer of olive oil. Gently wash the squash blossoms and place them on a towel to dry. Remove the pistils with a sharp knife (be careful not to damage the flower). Place all the goat chèvre into a small Ziploc or sandwich bag. Press the cheese into one corner and tie the opening off tightly with a twist tie or a rubber band. Cut the tip of the corner off with scissors. Place the opening directly into each squash blossom and squeeze until half-filled with cheese. Place the stuffed squash blossoms on the sheet pan and lightly drizzle with olive oil. Bake for about 10 minutes. Goat chèvre may be substituted with vegan soft cheese.

KOHLRABI FRIES!

Preheat oven to 425°F. Peel kohlrabi. Slice into fries. Toss in olive oil, sea salt and black pepper, as well as any other desired seasoning. Bake for 20 minutes.

KALE, ROASTED RED PEPPER AND GOAT CHEESE POPOVERS

1 standard package of puff pastry sheets

1 bunch kale

2 tablespoons extra virgin olive oil

Pinch of sea salt

1 small jar roasted red peppers, chopped

1 8-ounce package of goat cheese, cut into 12 equal pieces

Thaw package of puff pastry sheets and cut into squares. Massage kale with olive oil and sea salt. Preheat oven to 400°F. Place a few teaspoons each of kale, red peppers and goat cheese on squares. Fold into a triangle and pinch closed with your fingertips, sealing with a little water. Brush with olive oil and place on a greased cookie sheet. Bake for 10 minutes on each side or until golden brown.

TURNIP MASH ON A BED OF BRAISED GREENS TOPPED WITH CARAMELIZED ONIONS

8 turnips, cut into cubes

3 eggs, beaten

2 cups cheddar cheese, shredded

1 pound greens (any of these: kale, chard, spinach, turnip tops
  and radish tops)

3 onions, sliced thin

6 cloves of garlic, minced

Turnips: Boil turnip cubes for 20 minutes or until tender. Replace boiled and mashed turnips for potatoes in your favorite mashed potato recipe. Mash turnips with a potato masher or in the food processor. Add eggs and cheddar cheese and stir well. Bake for 20 minutes at 400°F. Top with caramelized onions.

Braised greens: Sauté onions and garlic. Set half the mixture aside for topping the dish. Add greens, a splash of balsamic and salt and cook until tender.

When serving, top greens with mashed turnips. Garnish with carmelized onions and garlic.

Roasted Veggies

A simple way to use your harvest! Preheat oven to 425° F. Cut your veggies into 1-inch pieces. Coat with extra virgin olive oil, a pinch of salt and your favorite spices and herbs. Lay veggies in a single layer on a sheet pan. Bake for 25–30 minutes, flipping veggies halfway through.

Cook firm root veggies such as carrots and potatoes together and tender veggies such as peppers and squash together. (Tender veggies may only need 15 minutes depending on the oven.)

Roasted veggies make excellent additions to quesadillas, sandwiches, pizza, soups and stews. Freeze leftovers for later use.

Main Dishes

Radicchio Ravioli with Walnut Sauce

Stuff individual radicchio leaves with your favorite ravioli filling. I like to use goat cheese, pesto, Parmesan cheese, sun-dried tomato pesto, caramelized onions and fresh parsley. Fold them like packets, using the goat cheese to close them. Pan sear with olive oil and sliced onions. I like to top them with a white wine, butter and walnut sauce with fresh parsley.

Radicchio is a specialty Italian vegetable in the chicory family. Peel back the outer leaves to view its vibrant and beautiful center. Radicchio is great mixed into salads, grilled and sautéed. It has a unique bitter flavor so be sure to neutralize the intensity with something creamy. Radicchio is a nutrient-rich vegetable and a good source of dietary fiber, containing vitamins B6, C, E and K as well as iron, magnesium, phosphorus, zinc, copper, manganese and potassium, among others.

Homemade Polenta with Fire-roasted Chilies

One of my favorite dishes to make from scratch is polenta with kale, chard, spring onions and squash blossoms.

Preheat oven to 400°F. Follow a basic polenta recipe (corn grits) but add your favorite ingredients such as sun-dried tomatoes, or our favorite, fire-roasted green chilies. Coat a glass pie pan with a small amount of olive oil. Put polenta mixture in pie pan and bake for 15 minutes. Let cool and refrigerate. Place pie pan upside down on a large plate. Use a spatula to gently remove. Top with your favorite ingredients such as salsa verde.

SPINACH AND KALE POLENTA TOPPED WITH VEGETARIAN BROWN GRAVY AND CARAMELIZED ONIONS

Follow basic polenta (corn grits) recipe. Add chopped kale, spinach, fresh herbs, salt, garlic, chives and olive oil. Once polenta is cooked according to package directions, pour into a greased glass pie pan and press down. Let it set for 30 minutes. Flip it upside down onto an oven-safe plate. Finish with gravy and caramelized onions and reheat in the oven for 10 minutes before serving. Enjoy!

ROASTED BUTTERNUT SQUASH WITH LEMON BUTTER SAUCE

Preheat oven to 425°F. Cut butternut squash in half, lengthwise. Remove seeds (save to plant in your garden). Brush both sides with olive oil. Roast on a sheet pan for 15–20 minutes on each side until golden brown and semi-soft. Melt 1 stick of butter in a saucepan. Squeeze 1 lemon into the butter. Add a pinch of salt and stir well. Pour the lemon butter over the squash and serve hot.

GRILLED SQUASH WITH BBQ SAUCE

When it's in season, we like to use squash as a main course as much as possible. It's incredibly versatile. Serve it hot or cold, cooked or raw; it can be shredded, sliced, chopped, sautéed, boiled, broiled, steamed, puréed and much more.

Grilling is one of our favorite ways to prepare squash. Simply slice lengthwise, brush with extra virgin olive oil, sea salt, pepper and a pinch of Cajun seasoning if you like spicy. Grill for about 3–5 minutes on each side. Drizzle with organic BBQ sauce.

White "Chicken" Chili

    6 large summer squash
    Olive oil
    1 pound white beans
    1 pound kidney beans
    2 onions, chopped
    6 stalks celery, chopped
    6 small colorful sweet peppers
    Salt, pepper, cumin, garlic powder, smoked paprika and chili
        powder, to taste
    ½ cup half-and-half
    1 jar of green salsa
    1 cup shredded Monterey jack cheese

Preheat oven to 425°F. Cube squash, toss with olive oil and roast for 20 minutes. Cook beans. Cut veggies, then sauté them in olive oil with spices in a skillet. Combine beans, squash and veggies in a large pot and add half-and-half, green salsa and cheese. Simmer on low for 45 minutes to let flavors marry. Serve with blue corn tortilla chips, a dollop of sour cream and scallions.

Farmer Eric's Veggie Samosas

    3 cups garbanzo/fava flour (or gluten-free flour)
    2 tablespoons baking soda
    1 tablespoon sea salt
    1 tablespoon flax meal (ground flax seeds)
    ½ cup water
    ½ cup extra virgin olive oil

Preheat oven to 400°F. Combine dry ingredients well. Pour in wet ingredients and mix well. Use your hands to knead the dough until wet and thoroughly mixed. Roll dough into a ball. With a rolling pin, roll into a rectangle, about ¼ inch thick, on a lightly floured surface. Cut into 12–24 even squares (depending on desired samosa size).

Fill squares with 2 tablespoons of roasted veggies, grilled veggies, sautéed veggies, leftover curry, mashed potatoes and peas or whatever your heart desires!

With your finger, brush the edges of each square with a little water. Fold into a triangle, pressing the edges firmly together to seal. Bake for 15–20 minutes or until golden.

WILD GREENS SPANAKOPITA WITH WILD ONION DIPPING SAUCE

(This recipe was originally published in *Feast Magazine*.)

This dish is sure to entice the beginning forager and get the taste buds accustomed to wild foods. Integrating them into your diet through tasty dishes and then slowly transitioning to the foods in their bare form is a way I have found to be enjoyable. Once a forager, always a forager.

Spanakopita — an authentic Greek pie that combines crispy layers of golden brown phyllo dough with spinach, cheeses and herbs — can be slightly altered to use wild greens. Often fibrous, they are easily cut with kitchen scissors.

> ½ cup extra virgin olive oil
> 1 16-ounce package phyllo dough
> 2 cups wild greens (¾ cup dandelion, ¾ cup plantain, ¼ cup
>   chickweed and ¼ cup red clover leaves), washed and
>   chopped finely
> 2 cups spinach, washed and chopped finely
> 3 cloves garlic, minced
> ¼ cup chopped roasted red pepper
> 3 tablespoons minced wild onions (or cut finely with kitchen
>   scissors)
> 1 cup feta cheese crumbles (optional)
> Pinch of sea salt
> Pinch of cracked black pepper
> Pinch each of thyme, dill and parsley
> 1 stick butter

Preheat oven to 425°F. Grease an 11x 17-inch glass baking dish, including the sides, with 1 to 2 tablespoons of olive oil. Remove phyllo dough from the package and unroll to thaw. Place a damp towel over it to prevent drying. Heat 4 tablespoons olive oil in a large skillet. Add all greens, garlic, roasted red pepper, wild onions, herbs, salt and pepper. Sauté for about 15 minutes on low-medium heat or until the greens are wilted and tender. Set mixture aside.

In a small saucepan, melt the butter. Add the remaining olive oil and stir well.

Assembling spanakopita is quite tedious and rather time-consuming, but the end result makes it worthwhile. Traditionally, spanakopitas are individually wrapped. However, the quicker method is to layer individual sheets with the greens mixture in a large baking dish. Place the first layer of phyllo at the bottom of the greased dish. With a pastry brush, spread the butter/oil mixture over the sheet. Add another layer of phyllo and brush completely with the butter/oil mixture. Repeat until 12 sheets of phyllo are in the baking dish. Add half of the greens mixture and sprinkle half of the feta cheese crumbles evenly over the phyllo. Repeat the process: add 12 sheets of individually buttered phyllo sheets followed by the remaining greens mixture and feta cheese. Add the remaining sheets of phyllo, individually buttering each layer.

Brush an extra coat of the butter/oil mixture to the top layer and bake for 15 minutes or until golden brown. Watch closely so that the spanakopita does not burn. Cut into 8 squares or 16 triangles.

Serve spanakopita as a side dish to a Greek-inspired meal or as the main attraction served with soup and salad.

Wild Onion Dipping Sauce

1 8-ounce package goat chèvre
½ cup plain yogurt
½ cucumber, chopped fine
⅛ cup minced wild onions
2 tablespoons dill, fresh or dry
1 teaspoon sea salt

Soften goat cheese in a bowl. Whip together the yogurt and goat cheese until smooth. Add the remaining ingredients and stir well.

Spicy Sweet Potato Latkes

2 cups shredded sweet potatoes
1 onion
2 poblano peppers, thinly sliced
½ cup panko crumbs
2 eggs
Salt to taste

Combine all ingredients in a bowl. Drop spoonfuls into hot oil and cook on each side for 2 minutes or until golden brown.

Sweet Treats

RAW BLUEBERRY MACAROONS

(Makes 12 macaroons)

>2 cups unsweetened shredded coconut
>½ cup raisins or pitted dates
>1 cup nuts
>⅛ cup maple syrup or honey
>1 cup frozen or fresh wild blueberries

In a food processor, blend all ingredients except blueberries until fine. Add blueberries and blend until smooth, or you are able to form balls. Make 12 balls, roll them in shredded coconut and refrigerate for 1 hour... or devour immediately if you can't wait.

LIZ'S SEASONAL FRUIT SALAD WITH HONEY MINT DRESSING

Chop 2 sprigs of fresh mint (apple mint is best). Add ¼ cup of honey and stir well. Mix into any fruit salad. Seasonal fruits are great. I like to combine peaches with cantaloupe and watermelon because I can buy them locally in the summer. I do enjoy bananas in a fruit salad though, so I buy organic bananas.

Edible flowers make a beautiful garnish.

Easy and Impressive Dishes

RATATOUILLE

A family favorite, ratatouille is fun to make and delicious. From start to finish, it takes about an hour to make.

>3 potatoes
>1 small eggplant
>1 zucchini
>1 summer squash
>1 pepper
>6 mushrooms
>1 to 2 jars pasta sauce
>1 cup shaved Parmesan

Preheat oven to 400°F. Slice veggies (I use a food processor to slice the potatoes, squash and eggplant.). In a lightly greased baking dish, arrange ingredients, in the following order: potatoes, eggplant, sauce, cheese, squash, mushrooms, peppers, sauce and cheese. Bake for 30 minutes.

Other Simple Ideas

HONEY-GLAZED ROSEMARY TURNIPS SAUTÉED IN BROWN BUTTER

> 6 turnips
> ½ stick butter
> 1 sprig fresh rosemary
> 6 tablespoons honey

Cut turnips into thin slices and then quarter the slices. In a large skillet, melt the butter and sauté slices until golden. Add fresh rosemary and honey. Sauté until the turnips are caramelized.

PAN-SEARED TURNIP GREENS AND ONIONS WITH RED WINE VINEGAR AND BUTTER

> 1 medium onion
> Turnip greens from 6 turnips
> ½ stick butter
> 4 garlic cloves, minced
> ⅛ cup red wine vinegar

Cut onion into thin slices. Chop turnip greens into small pieces. In a large skillet, melt butter and sauté sliced onions until golden. Add minced garlic and turnip greens and sauté for 8–10 minutes. Add red wine vinegar and simmer on low for 2 minutes.

GARLIC SCAPE ROASTED POTATOES

> 12 potatoes
> 3 garlic scapes, minced
> 4 tablespoons extra virgin olive oil
> 1 pinch each salt and pepper

Preheat oven to 425°F. Cut potatoes into 1-inch cubes and toss in olive oil with garlic scapes. Roast for 20–25 minutes.

Carrots can be planted in the Midwest in early spring for summer harvest, but they can also be grown all summer long for early autumn harvest. They are highly nutritious and have a unique earthy flavor like other root vegetables. The carrots cultivated along the Mississippi River and in the river valleys are packed with flavor. There is something so satisfying about pulling vibrant orange carrots out of the rich dark soil after sowing the seed, weeding, watering and waiting.

Carrots are my husband's favorite crop: "The reward of growing carrots is truly remarkable. Although it seems to be a long wait from seed to harvest, the carrot root develops its flavor and crunch from the cool spring rains and its size as the seasons change."

In this delicious spice cake recipe, carrots share the spotlight with calendula flowers. The moist cake and the shredded carrots offer a neutral base to indulge in the distinctive texture of the calendula flower, which can be eaten and surprisingly enjoyed whole. The Irish whiskey-soaked raisins give a nice finishing touch to the richness of this early autumn dessert.

THREE-TIERED CARROT CALENDULA CAKE WITH HONEY CREAM CHEESE AND 4 HANDS CAST IRON BROWN FROSTING

4 cups all purpose flour

1 tablespoon baking soda

2½ tablespoons baking powder

3 tablespoons ground cinnamon

1 teaspoon allspice

½ teaspoon ground cloves

1 tablespoon ground nutmeg

1 teaspoon ground ginger

1 teaspoon salt

1 cup applesauce

1 stick butter (softened)

1 cup coconut oil (softened)

1 cup coconut sugar

1 cup honey

2 cups shredded carrots

¼ cup calendula petals (fresh or dried)

1 cup raisins soaked in ¼ cup Irish whiskey + ¾ cup milk +
1 tablespoon honey

1 teaspoon hot pepper flakes

1 tablespoon sriracha hot sauce

5 eggs

1 cup vanilla almond milk

2 tablespoons pure vanilla extract

1 tablespoon apple cider vinegar

Preheat oven to 375°F.

In a large mixing bowl, whisk together the flour, baking soda, baking powder, cinnamon, allspice, ground cloves, ground nutmeg, ground ginger and salt.

In a medium bowl, combine the coconut sugar, applesauce, honey, butter and coconut oil. Blend together using an electric mixer. Add the eggs, one at a time just until the mixture is whipped together.

In a small bowl, beat the apple cider vinegar and the vanilla extract into the almond milk. Add this to the sugar and egg mixture and stir well. Add the shredded carrots, calendula petals, raisins (with the soaking mixture), the hot pepper flakes and the sriracha and stir well.

Fold the wet ingredients into the dry ingredients. Lightly grease 3 pie pans, one slightly larger than the other (Glass Pyrex bowls work well; aluminum cake pans will work, just as long as you have three tiers).

Bake for 30 minutes or until a toothpick poked into the middle of the cake comes out clean.

Calendula, revered as a favorite in the wonderful world of edible flowers, make a gorgeous decoration to cakes and cupcakes. They are a gem in the culinary world; the petals make a stunning jelly, and it is a main component in floral herbal teas. Calendula is also highly medicinal and has been used since ancient times to accelerate healing both internally and topically.

Calendula flowers, native perennials to the Mediterranean climate, can be easily grown in the Midwest throughout late spring, summer and fall, appearing in various shades of orange and yellow. Their sweet nuttiness pairs nicely with farm-fresh carrots, especially when crafted into a carrot spice cake.

Gluten Free Option

> 1 package Namaste Foods Gluten Free Spice Cake Mix
>   (26 ounces)
> 2 cups shredded carrots
> 1 cup applesauce
> 1 cup raisins
> ¼ cup Irish whiskey
> ¾ cup milk
> 1 tablespoon honey
> 2 tablespoons cinnamon
> 1 teaspoon hot pepper flakes
> 1 squirt sriracha hot sauce

Soak raisins in whiskey, milk and honey. Follow cake mix instructions and fold in the remaining ingredients. Bake according to package directions.

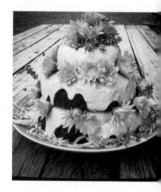

Honey Cream Cheese and 4 Hands Cast Iron Oatmeal Brown Frosting

Using chocolate malt and roasted barley to give this beer a cast-iron backbone, 4 Hands oatmeal brown beer pours a dark mahogany with aromas of dark chocolate and coffee.

> 1 8 ounce package organic cream cheese (softened)
> ½ cup honey
> 1 tablespoon cinnamon
> ¼ cup 4 hands Cast Iron Oatmeal Brown Beer

Mix frosting ingredients in a food processor until smooth.

Assemble cake with largest tier on the bottom. Stack the remaining tiers and glaze cake by pouring frosting in a spiral motion over the three tiers. Decorate with edible calendula flowers.

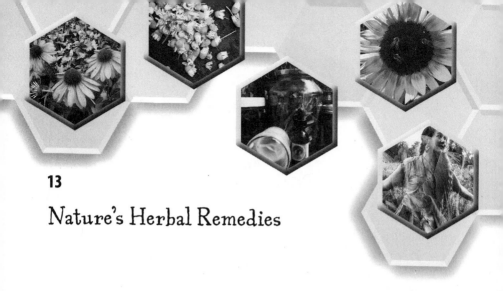

13

Nature's Herbal Remedies

ERBAL ELIXIRS are one of my favorite ways to use herbs. They really embody the essence of an herb through flavor, aroma, energetics and the effect the herb has on the mind, body and spirit. Historically, herbal elixirs were used medicinally, as a pleasant way to treat a variety of ailments.

Essentially, herbal elixirs involve steeping medicinal herbs in honey or maple syrup, sometimes combining them with brandy or other alcohol, or fermenting them, such as medicinal meads.

Basic Herbal Elixir

Simply combine equal parts of herbal honey and herbal tincture. Fill a pint jar with medicinal herbs of your choice. Pour ⅓ pint of honey over the herbs, covering them all the way. Pour brandy over herbs and honey to fill the jar. Place a plastic lid on the jar and shake well. Place on a small plate to prevent leakage. Store in a dark cupboard for about a month. Strain the herbs. Enjoy the elixir 2 ounces at a time. Keep refrigerated to preserve longevity.

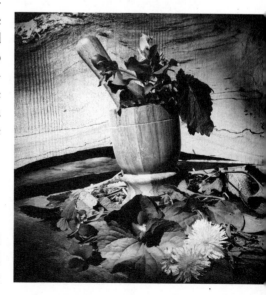

Herbal-infused Waters and Cold Herbal Infusions

Cucumber Mint Water

Being out in the sun for extended lengths leaves us dehydrated and thirsty. I try to keep the farm crew hydrated with refreshing infused herbal water creations such as cucumber mint, strawberry fennel dandelion and lemon balm with citrus fruit. The one that cools us off the most is cucumber mint. Cucumbers are loaded with B vitamins and electrolytes. Mint has a cooling effect on the body and is good for temperature regulation. Mint also has antiviral properties and has a calming effect on the nervous system. Mint has been used throughout history to treat such ailments as headaches, liver complaints, digestive problems and colds.

Fill a 1-quart Mason jar with purified water. Add one sliced cucumber and 3 sprigs of mint. Let the cucumber and mint infuse in the water for at least 30 minutes.

Raspberry, Raspberry Leaf and Red Clover

Red raspberry leaf and red clover both help to promote women's health, to tone the uterus and to reduce menstrual cramps, symptoms of PMS and hot flashes during menopause.

Fill a 1-quart Mason jar with purified water.

Add 4 tablespoons of fresh red raspberry leaves, 2 tablespoons of red clover and ½ cup of raspberries.

Strawberry Fennel

Strawberries are loaded with antioxidants and high in vitamin C and manganese. Fennel is nutrient-rich and aids in digestion and stomach upsets.

Fill a 1-quart Mason jar with purified water. Add 3 chopped strawberries and 3 sprigs of fresh fennel. Infuse for at least 30 minutes.

Strawberry Dandelion

Strawberries are loaded with antioxidants and high in vitamin C and manganese. Dandelions are vitamin- and nutrient-rich, boosting immunity.

Fill a 1-quart Mason jar with purified water. Add 3 chopped strawberries and 10 dandelions. Infuse for at least 30 minutes.

Blackberry Sage

Blackberries are rich in antioxidants, minerals and vitamins. They are an excellent source of vitamin C. Sage is vitamin- and nutrient-rich and is a good lung tonic.

Fill a 1-quart Mason jar with purified water. Add ½ cup of fresh blackberries and 1 sprig of fresh sage. Infuse for at least 30 minutes.

Lavender Mixed Berry

Soothing and refreshing, rich in vitamins and minerals, antioxidant-rich.

Fill a 1-quart Mason jar with purified water, mixed berries and lavender. Infuse for at least 30 minutes.

Lavender Chamomile

Soothing and relaxing.

Fill a 1-quart Mason jar with purified water. Add 2 sprigs of lavender and 10 chamomile flowers. Let the herbs infuse for about an hour before enjoying.

St. John's Wort

Uplifting and mood-enhancing.

Fill a 1-quart Mason jar with purified water. Add 1 ounce of fresh St. John's wort, leaves and flowers. Infuse herbs for about an hour before enjoying.

Purple Basil, Apple Mint, Echinacea, Tulsi

Uplifting, immune building, cooling, soothing, refreshing, overall health and well-being tonic.

Fill a 1-quart Mason jar with purified water. Add 1 sprig each of purple basil, apple mint and tulsi. Add one echinacea flower or 1 tablespoon of echinacea root. Let the herbs infuse for about an hour before enjoying.

Lemon Balm Herbal Lemonade

Lemon balm produces a very delightful herbal lemonade. Makes 2.5 gallons

Infuse 1 bunch of mint and 1 small bunch of lemon balm in 1 gallon of purified water and let steep for 30 to 60 minutes.

Add ½ dropper-full of liquid stevia extract. Add 1 cup of organic lemon juice concentrate. Add 3 sliced organic lemons. Add ½ bag of ice. Garnish with fresh herbs (mint, lemon balm, rosemary) and edible flowers. Add echinacea and St. John's wort.

Nutrient-rich lemonade is high in vitamins and minerals, helps to cool the body and boost immunity and is an uplifting tonic.

Home Apothecary 101

Most of the supplies needed for your own herbal apothecary can be grown yourself, purchased online through Mountain Rose Herbs or Starwest Botanicals, or at your local herb store or natural foods store.

Hot Infusions
Tea

"From its humble beginnings in the Himalayan foothills of Southeast Asia, the salubrious tea plant has been traded by humans to every nook and cranny of the globe, and adopted by every people under the sun. Long before igniting the American War of Independence, it abetted the poets of China in their greatest achievements. It has burrowed itself to the core of the Japanese soul, solaced many a weary Tibetan yak herder, fueled the midnight cogitations of Britain's great inventors, and offered untold numbers of Russian peasants with a path to sobriety. Through the centuries, it has provided a safe, stimulating beverage that played a crucial role in reducing human epidemics and making habitation in crowded, bustling cities possible. In the modern world, it marks the day's rhythm for hundreds and millions of people, from the Koryaks of the Kamchatka Peninsula in Russia to the Samburu pastoralists in Northern Kenya. It is precisely the epic nature of tea's odyssey that has always made its history so difficult to write. With its botanical, medical, religious, cultural, economic, anthropological, social and political dimensions, with its roots in antiquity and utter unconcern for distances and linguistic divides, the task of gathering its many strands into a single story for the general reader has always proved daunting for authors, whether from the West or the East."

— Excerpt from *The True History of Tea*
by Victor H. Mair and Erling Hoh

Hot infusions are soothing, warming and comforting during winter months. Herbs can be steeped for 5–10 minutes to extract the active constituents and the medicinal benefits from the herb. Leaves and flowers require less time to steep than roots and bark.

Herbal Tea Blends

Cold and flu support tea: thyme, oregano, sage, rosemary, cloves, cinnamon bark, ginger, mullein, stevia leaf, lemon and honey

Floral energy tea: red clover flowers, calendula flowers, chrysanthemum flowers, echinacea petals, rose hips, lemon balm, red raspberry leaf, nettles

Digestion tea: ginger root, peppermint leaf, basil leaf, and chamomile flowers

Rest and relax tea: chamomile and valerian root

Stress relief tea: kava kava, chamomile flowers, spearmint, passionflower herb, rose petals, lavender flowers and cinnamon bark

Immune builder tea: echinacea, goldenseal, red clover blossoms, nettle leaf, pau d'arco bark, sage leaf, St. John's wort and ginger root

Headache relief tea: peppermint leaves and lavender flowers

Making Your Own Herbal Tea

Preparing your own herbal tea is fun and cost-effective. You can grow most of the tea plants yourself. Keep your dried tea blends in a Mason jar.

I make roughly six cups of tea at a time in a six-cup glass Pyrex measuring dish. It can also be made in a medium pot. I boil the water and remove from heat. I place my herbs in the glass measuring cup and cover with the hot water for five to ten minutes. I strain the herbs and add honey. What my family doesn't drink, I refrigerate for later use. A fine mesh stainless steel strainer works great to strain the herb. For individual servings use a stainless steel tea ball that latches. Tea balls are designed to steep loose herbs for individual servings.

Other Tea Ideas

Buy "tea bags" and fill them with the blend of your choice. Iron the tea bags shut and store them in a jar or decorative tin.

Teas make excellent gifts. Package them beautifully with a small jar of local honey. If it is for a very special person, include a tea set.

You may purchase dried stevia leaf and add it to your tea blend to naturally sweeten it.

HERBAL-INFUSED OILS OR HERBAL OIL INFUSION

Herbal oil infusions are used topically for dry skin or to heal blemishes. They can also be used to make lip balm, first-aid salve or other healing salves. Making an herbal oil infusion simply involves soaking herbs or flowers in a jar of oil, then straining the herb to use the oil.

Mason jar with lid

1 cup dried herbs or 3 cups fresh herbs (dandelion, calendula, echinacea, plantain and lemon balm)

2 cups carrier oil (grapeseed oil, extra virgin olive oil, sunflower oil, sweet almond oil or apricot oil)

3 capsules vitamin E oil

Pack your herbs in a large glass jar, cover with oil and add vitamin E capsules, leaving an inch at the top. Shake vigorously. Seal the jar and leave it in a warm, slightly sunny place for 2 weeks, shaking daily.

Pour into a clean glass jar, straining through cheesecloth. Squeeze as much oil through the bag, and pour into clean dark glass bottles.

Seal the bottles and store in the refrigerator for up to 3 months.

First-Aid Salve

This great general-purpose healing salve will make about 10 ounces.

> 2 cups of your herbal-infused oil (comfrey, chickweed, calendula, echinacea, plantain, lemon balm, dandelion)
> 1 ounce grated or chopped beeswax
> 3 vitamin E capsules of at least 400 units (this is your preservative)
> 10 drops of lavender essential oil
> Cheesecloth
> Double boiler or 2 pots (one that fits inside of the other)
> Glass measuring cup
> Large spoon
> Stainless steel container with a narrow pouring spout
> Baby food jars or tins
> Labels or a permanent marker

Place your herbal oil infusion in the top pot of your double boiler on a burner or on the stovetop. Very GENTLY heat the oil mix on low.

Add your beeswax in the top pot of your double boiler on a burner or on the stove-top. Stir until it's completely melted and blended.

Place your Herbal Oil Infusion & vitamin E oil in with the melted beeswax and stir well until it dissolves. Very GENTLY heat the oil mix on low. Remove from heat and let cool.

Pour into a wide mouth jar or several small jars. As it cools, the mixture will become semi-solid and the perfect salve consistency.

First-aid salve may be used in place of double or triple antibiotic ointment. It helps to heal minor cuts, scrapes and burns. It also helps with bruises, dry skin, joint and muscle pain and even arthritis pain.

Poison Ivy Relief Salve

> 2 cups oil infused with fresh or dried jewelweed

Follow recipe for first-aid salve, replacing the herb-infused oil with this.

TINCTURE MAKING

Tincture making is an ancient art that has been passed down through generations, usually from mother to daughter, around the globe.

Tinctures involve soaking herbs in a liquid — typically vodka, brandy, apple cider vinegar or vegetable glycerin — to extract the medicinal properties of the herbs. Alcohol tends to have a long shelf life so the tincture will last several years. Vinegar and glycerin tinctures have a shorter shelf life and may need to be refrigerated. The liquid used in tincture making is known as the menstruum.

The standard ratio for fresh herbs in tincture making is 1 part fresh herb to 2 parts menstruum. For example, for a single herb St. John's wort tincture, for every ounce of fresh St. John's wort used, you would need 2 ounces of menstruum. The standard ratio for dried herbs is 1 part dried herbs to 5 parts menstruum.

Typically the herb will rise to the top of the jar, above the liquid surface. To prevent this from happening, weigh down your herbs with a crystal (be sure to sanitize the crystal first).

For advanced tincture-making, 190-proof organic alcohol works best. Different herbs require varying concentrations of alcohol.

SIMPLE TINCTURE

Herbs and flowers of your choice
Mason jar with lid
Alcohol (organic vodka or brandy)

Label your jar with contents and date. Fill jar ¾ of the way full with herbs. Fill jar halfway with alcohol. Add water, leaving 1 inch at the top of the jar. Be sure your herbs are covered. If they are not, tamp them down with a spoon. Shake vigorously for 1–2 minutes.

Store in a dark, cool, dry place. Shake daily. Medicine will be ready in 2 weeks and will last up to 1 year.

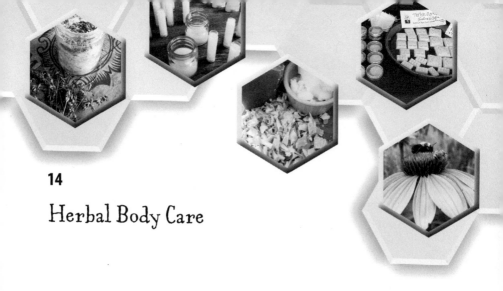

14

Herbal Body Care

W HEN IT COMES TO HERBAL BODY CARE, I use the same set of standards for checking food labels. If I can't pronounce it or don't know what it is, it's probably not a good idea to put it in or on my body. For me, transitioning to homemade herbal body care was easy. Lotion, body wash, shampoo and conditioner were really the only products I bought. I didn't wear makeup. I didn't use hair spray or shaving gel or all the other dozens of products marketed toward young and impressionable women. I was more of a tomboy, I suppose. But even for women who do rely on store-bought beauty products, making the transition is actually quite easy. Coconut oil alone could replace several beauty care products. It makes a wonderful lotion, a mouth rinse to fight cavities, and it makes the hair shiny and healthy, just to name a few benefits.

The following recipes are easy and cost-effective. You could either prepare the full batches or make them with your friends, splitting the costs of the raw ingredients and sharing the various products.

When choosing scents, think in terms of which scents or tastes speak to you. For a mint flavor or aroma, use peppermint and spearmint essential oils; for chai flavor or aroma, use small amounts of cinnamon, nutmeg, ginger and clove essential oils; for a citrus blend, use grapefruit and orange. Purchase pure essential oils online or at your local health food store. It is best to get pure food or cosmetic-grade essential oils.

LIP BALM

> 1 cup coconut oil or other solid carrier oil
>
> ½ cup hempseed oil
>
> 2 tablespoons vitamin E oil
>
> 1½ ounces beeswax (or ¾ ounce candelilla wax and ½ ounce soy
>   wax for vegan lip balm)
>
> ¼ ounce cocoa butter
>
> Pure essential oils
>
> Double boiler or 2 pots, one smaller than the other
>
> Small stainless steel pitcher with spout
>
> Approximately 50 lip balm tubes or tins (available online under
>   the title "eco-friendly lip balm tubes")

Have all ingredients available and ready. Set up lip balm tubes upright with enough space between each tube to grab and fill.

Pour about 2–3 inches of water into the bottom pot of a double boiler, depending on the size of your heating element. Once the water boils, turn heat to low.

Place beeswax (or candelilla wax and soy wax for vegan lip balm) and cocoa butter into the smaller stainless steel pot and stir frequently until completely melted. Add coconut oil, hempseed oil and vitamin E oil. Stir well until mixture is liquid again.

Turn heat off. With a potholder, remove the pot with the mixture and pour it into the small stainless steel pitcher with the narrow spout. Stir in 10–15 drops of essential oils.

Immediately pour mixture into the lip balm tubes. A pitcher with a narrow pour spout works fairly well if you pour slowly. Otherwise, use a stainless steel funnel.

Let the tubes sit until they harden. Once they harden, put the caps on, wipe them with a clean damp cloth and label.

LOTION

½ cup coconut oil
¼ cup shea butter
¼ cup cocoa butter
1 cup emulsifying wax
2 tablespoons vitamin E oil
4 cups hot water
¼ teaspoons citric acid
Pure essential oils (pick gentle ones such as lavender)

Melt oils, butter and wax together in a double boiler on low. Put mixture and hot water into large stainless steel bowl. Mix for one minute using an electric mixer or whip by hand. Store in a baby food jar with tight-fitting lid.

SUNSCREEN

½ cup coconut oil
¼ cup shea butter
¼ cup cocoa butter
1 cup emulsifying wax
4 tablespoons beeswax
2 tablespoons vitamin E oil
4 cups hot water
¼ teaspoons citric acid
10 tablespoons zinc oxide
10 tablespoons aloe vera gel
Pure essential oils (gentle ones such as lavender or eucalyptus)

Melt oils, butters and waxes together in a double boiler on low heat. Put melted mixture, hot water and citric acid into a large stainless steel mixing bowl. Mix for 1 minute using an electric mixer, or whip by hand.

After the mixture cools, add zinc oxide and aloe vera gel. Add more if you would like to increase SPF. One tablespoon of each will increase the SPF by 5.

For an insect repellent component, add 15 drops of citronella essential oil, 5 drops of eucalyptus essential oil, 10 drops of lemongrass essential oil and 10 drops of lavender essential oil.

Store in baby food jars with tight fitting-lids.

Vegan option: replace beeswax with candelilla and soy wax.

Insect Repellent Spray

1 gallon purified water
20 drops citronella essential oil
10 drops eucalyptus essential oil
15 drops lemongrass essential oil
10 drops lavender essential oil

Remove and discard 2 cups of water from a gallon of purified water. Add essential oils. Place lid on container and shake vigorously for 1 minute.

Fill spray bottles with a funnel, shaking before each pour.

Label spray bottles. Shake well before each use.

Body Wash

1 cup water
2 cups liquid castile soap
4 tablespoons melted coconut oil
10–15 drops lavender essential oil or essential oils of your choice

Never use clove oil or oregano oil directly on the skin as they will burn. If you choose peppermint essential oil, use only half of the suggested number of drops. To be safe, stick to gentle essential oils such as lavender and rosemary. Small amounts of tea tree or other safe essential oils can be used as well.

Whisk all ingredients together in a measuring cup. Using a funnel, fill a reused body wash or squirt bottle. Be sure to label. Use 1 or 2 squeezes per wash.

Invigorating Shampoo

1 cup water
½ cup liquid castile soap
8 tablespoons apple cider vinegar
1 tablespoon coconut or calendula oil
10 drops peppermint essential oil
10 drops lavender essential oil
10 drops rosemary essential oil

Whisk together all ingredients in a measuring cup. Funnel into reused shampoo bottle. Be sure to label. Use 1 or 2 squeezes per shampoo.

Natural Mint Toothpaste

> 6 tablespoons baking soda
> 1 tablespoon Celtic sea salt
> 5–10 drops peppermint or spearmint essential oil
> 1 tablespoon water

Mix together ingredients in a small plastic container with lid. Be sure to label. Use ½ teaspoon per cleaning. Use within 3 months.

Spearmint Mouthwash

> 1 cup water
> ½ cup vodka
> 10–15 drops peppermint or spearmint essential oil
> 2 teaspoons aloe vera gel (optional)
> 5 teaspoons liquid vegetable glycerin (optional)

Bring water and vodka to a boil and then let cool. Add 10–15 drops of peppermint or spearmint essential oil and mix well. If you like, add aloe vera gel and liquid vegetable glycerin. Transfer to a recycled mouthwash container and shake well before each use. Be sure to label. Use 1 capful per rinse.

Bath Salts

Simply combine sea salt, lavender or chamomile flowers and a pinch of baking soda in a quart or pint jar. Add 10–15 drops lavender essential oil.

Salt and Sugar Scrubs

Combine equal parts olive oil and sea salt or sugar as well as 20 to 30 drops of essential oils of peppermint or lavender, or other pure essential oil safe for topical application. Stir well and pour into a jar with a secure lid.

It is easy to create beautiful handcrafted artisan soaking salts and exfoliating scrubs. These also make excellent gifts when packaged nicely with homemade labels.

Deodorant

> 1 cup coconut oil
> 1 tablespoon vitamin E oil
> ½ ounce beeswax
> 1 ounce shea butter
> 40 drops lavender essential oil

Mix coconut oil, vitamin E oil, beeswax and shea butter together in a double boiler. Let cool. Stir in essential oils. Store in small recycled jars (baby food size) jars with tight-fitting lids.

Natural Baby Wipes

> Medium stack of heavy-duty organic cloths (30)
> 2 cups water
> ½ cup aloe vera juice
> 2 tablespoons apple cider vinegar
> 2 tablespoons calendula oil or vitamin E oil
> 1 tablespoons liquid castile soap
> 2 drops lavender essential oil

Whisk all ingredients together in a large mixing bowl. Gently press down cloths into liquid so it is all absorbed. Place wet wipes in a reused wipe box with lid. Be sure to label.

Diaper Ointment

> 1 cup coconut oil (infused with ⅛ cup dried calendula flowers,
> ⅛ cup chamomile flowers and 5 plantain leaves)
> ¾ cup shea butter
> 1 tablespoon vitamin E oil
> 15 drops lavender essential oil
> 1 teaspoon non-nano zinc oxide

Infuse coconut oil with flowers and plantain on low heat for 20 minutes. Strain. Mix coconut oil and shea butter together in the top of a double boiler. Let cool. Stir in essential oils and zinc oxide. Store in recycled shallow jars with tight-fitting lids.

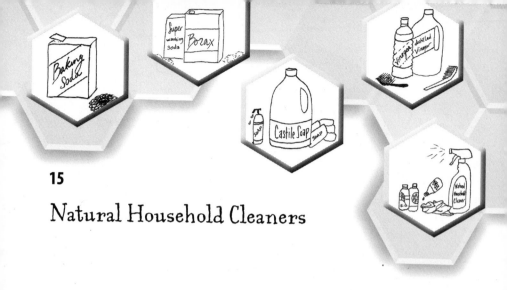

15

Natural Household Cleaners

HARSH CHEMICAL CLEANERS are harmful to the environment and toxic to our bodies. Some cause acute problems such as skin or respiratory irritation, watery eyes or chemical burns, while others are associated with chronic or long-term effects such as cancer. The most acutely dangerous cleaning products are corrosive drain cleaners, oven cleaners and acidic toilet bowl cleaners, according to Philip Dickey of the Washington Toxics Coalition:

> Corrosive chemicals can cause severe burns on eyes, skin and, if ingested, on the throat and esophagus. Ingredients with high acute toxicity include chlorine bleach and ammonia, which produce fumes that are highly irritating to eyes, nose, throat and lungs, and should not be used by people with asthma or lung or heart problems.

A few safe and simple ingredients such as liquid castile soap, water, baking soda, vinegar and lemon juice aided by a little elbow grease can tackle most household cleaning needs. These ingredients are eco-friendly and affordable. It is a myth that we need harsh chemical cleaners to do our dirty work; natural cleaners are just as effective for the majority of all cleaning tasks.

Natural Cleansers Are Abundant!

Vinegar is affordable and eco-friendly. It is acidic and helps remove bacteria, mildew, mold and grease, and neutralize odors.

Baking soda is very affordable and also eco-friendly. It helps to clean and scour tough surfaces, neutralize odors and can be used as laundry detergent.

Lemon has antibacterial, antiseptic and antimicrobial properties. Lemon essential oil, fresh lemon and lemon juice concentrate are all effective in cleaning.

Cornstarch can be used to clean windows and shampoo carpets and rugs.

Castile soap, an olive oil-based soap, can be used to make your own liquid dish soap, body wash and laundry detergent. Made from plant oils plus lye, it is eco-friendly and biodegradable.

Essential Oils and Their Properties

⊚ Cinnamon essential oil: antiseptic and antibacterial

⊚ Eucalyptus essential oil: antiseptic and pesticide

⊚ Geranium essential oil: antibacterial

⊚ Lavender essential oil: antibacterial, antifungal

⊚ Lemon essential oil: antibacterial, antiseptic and antimicrobial

⊚ Lemongrass essential oil: antiseptic and insecticidal

⊚ Oregano essential oil: antibacterial

⊚ Peppermint essential oil: antiseptic

⊚ Rosemary essential oil: antiseptic

⊚ Sage essential oil: antiseptic

⊚ Tea tree essential oil: antiseptic and antibacterial

⊚ Thyme essential oil: antiseptic and antibiotic

ANTIBACTERIAL HAND WIPES

1 roll of eco-friendly paper towels (such as Seventh Generation) or a stack of fabric scraps

3 cups water

1 tall circular wipes container or other plastic cylinder with lid

3 tablespoons natural shampoo or liquid castile soap

2 tablespoons hydrogen peroxide

10 drops lavender essential oil

10 drops tea tree essential oil

Cut the roll of paper towels in half with large scissors or sharp knife. Whisk the wet ingredients together in a large bowl. Pour about half of the mixture into the container. Slowly and carefully place the half roll of paper towels into the container. Pour the remaining mixture gently over the paper towels. Remove the cardboard center by firmly pressing the paper towels down and pulling the cardboard tube out. The hand wipes will stay good for about 2 months.

NATURAL ANTIBACTERIAL MULTI-SURFACE WIPES

2½ cups hot water (boiled, then cooled)
½ cup Simple Green cleaner or ½ cup vinegar
30 drops tea tree essential oil
20 drops lavender essential oil
1 roll of strong, durable eco-friendly paper towels cut in half, or a
    stack of fabric scraps
2 airtight cylinder or rectangle containers (diaper wipe
    containers and large coffee canisters work well)

Mix water, Simple Green (or vinegar) and essential oils in a large bowl. Cut the roll of paper towels in half with large scissors or sharp knife. Place each ½ roll (cut side down) in separate airtight cylinder or rectangle containers that will completely cover the roll. Pour the mixture over the paper towels. Remove the cardboard center by firmly pressing the paper towels down and pulling the cardboard tube out. Pull the first paper towel from the center. The wipes should spiral out easily. You can also use a stack of reusable cloths.

Natural All-purpose Cleaning Sprays

The following four recipes can be made directly in a spray bottle. Be sure to label them.

Works well on glass. Mix 2 parts water with 1 part distilled vinegar. Add 10–20 drops lavender essential oil.

Works well on hard-to-clean surfaces. Mix 2 cups water with 2 teaspoons castile soap, 10–20 drops lavender essential oil and 10–20 drops tea tree essential oil.

General all-purpose spray. Mix 1 cup water with 10–20 drops lavender essential oil and 10–15 drops peppermint essential oil.

General all-purpose spray, works well on glass. Mix 2 cups purified water with 3 tablespoons lemon juice, 1 tablespoon vinegar, and 10–20 drops tea tree essential oil. Be sure to label. Use 1 or 2 sprays per cleaning.

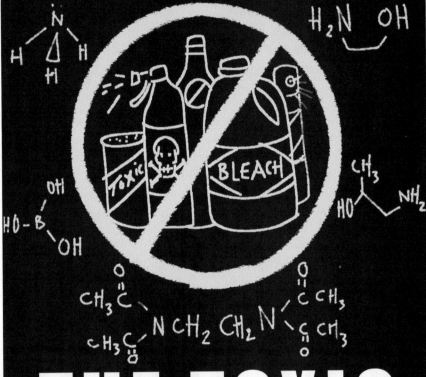

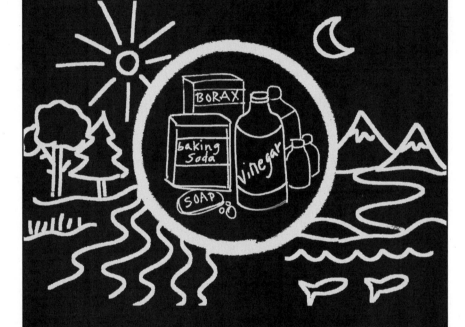

NATURAL DISH SOAP

½ cup castile soap

1 cup water

½ cup vinegar

1 teaspoon lemon juice

¼ cup soap base for suds (optional)

20 drops essential oil (lemon and lavender essential oils are
antibacterial and antifungal, and smell nice when combined)

Whisk together all ingredients in a measuring cup and funnel into an empty dish soap bottle. Shake well before each use. Be sure to label. Use 1 or 2 squirts per load of hand-washed dishes.

NATURAL GLASS CLEANER

2 cups purified water

4 tablespoons lemon juice

½ cup distilled vinegar

6 drops tea tree essential oil

Funnel all ingredients into a reused spray bottle. Be sure to label. Use 3 to 5 squirts per cleaning.

A trick my father taught me: instead of paper towels, use recycled black ink newspaper to clean glass. Simply ball it up, spray glass, wipe surface and viola. Streak-free shine!

NATURAL LIQUID LAUNDRY DETERGENT

2 bars of soap, finely grated with a cheese grater (Fels-Naptha
works well as do several smaller soap ends.

4 gallons hot water

2 cups super washing soda

2 cups borax

2 cups baking soda

20–50 drops essential oil (I use lavender, tea tree, lemon and
peppermint essential oils)

Melt grated soap in hot water in 5-gallon bucket and stir well. Add remaining ingredients and stir vigorously. You can leave the mixture in the bucket or transfer it to recycled liquid laundry detergent containers. Shake well before each use. Be sure to label. Use 1 cup per load. For extra scent, add 10 drops of your favorite essential oil to each load.

NATURAL LIQUID LAUNDRY DETERGENT WITH CASTILE SOAP

> 3 gallons water
> 4 cups liquid castile soap
> 1 cup distilled vinegar
> ½ cup vegetable glycerin
> 20 drops lavender essential oil
> 20 drops tea tree or lemon essential oil

Mix all ingredients together in a 5-gallon bucket. Transfer to recycled liquid laundry detergent containers if you wish. Be sure to label. Shake well before each use. Use ½ cup per medium load, or 1 cup per large load.

REUSABLE DRYER SHEETS

> 12 squares of scrap fabric (cut to the size of a standard dryer
> sheet). The more colorful the better so you can recognize
> them as dryer sheets
> 10–15 drops of your favorite essential oil

Simply place 10 to 15 drops of essential oil on 1 square and toss in dryer.

LAVENDER DRYER SACHETS

> 1 small muslin drawstring bag
> Dried lavender
> 2–3 drops lavender essential oil

Fill the muslin bag with the dried lavender and add the essential oil. Pull the drawstring tightly and knot it a few times. Simply keep the sachet in the dryer. The scent will last for about 20 loads.

NATURAL HAND SANITIZER

> ½ cup aloe vera gel
> ½ cup grain alcohol such as Everclear
> 10 drops tea tree or lemon essential oil
> 10 drops lavender essential oil

Whisk all ingredients together well in a bowl. Funnel ingredients into an empty plastic bottle. Be sure to label. Use 1 squeeze per use.

Natural Antibacterial Hand Soap

2 cups water

4 tablespoons liquid castile soap

2 teaspoons vegetable glycerin

10–20 drops lavender essential oil

10 drops tea tree or lemon essential oil

Wisk together all ingredients in a measuring cup. Funnel into a reused hand soap pump bottle. Be sure to label. Use 1 or 2 pumps per wash.

Kitchen and Bathroom Cleaners

Scrubbing Powder

2 cups baking soda

10–20 drops of lemon essential oil

Combine ingredients in a large bowl. Add to a reused bottle with a shaker lid. Use to scrub surfaces such as sinks and bathtubs. Be sure to label. Use 1 or 2 shakes per cleaning.

Natural Scouring Gel

1 cup natural dish soap or liquid castile soap

½ cup water

½ cup baking soda

15–20 drops lemon or tea tree essential oil

Whisk ingredients together in a bowl. Funnel into a squeeze container with lid. Be sure to label. Use 1 or 2 squeezes per cleaning.

Tub and Tile Cleaner

2 cups baking soda

2 cups water

1 cup liquid castile soap

4 tablespoons distilled white vinegar

15 drops tea tree essential oil

Whisk ingredients together in a bowl. Funnel into a squeeze container with lid. Be sure to label. Use 1 or 2 squeezes per cleaning.

TOILET CLEANER

2 cups borax
1 cup water
½ cup lemon juice
20 drops tea tree essential oil

Whisk ingredients together in a bowl. Funnel into a squeeze container with lid. Be sure to label. Use 1 or 2 squeezes per cleaning.

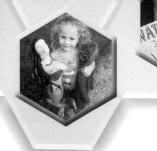
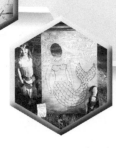
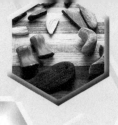

16

Create Your Own Gifts: Inexpensive DIY Gift Ideas for the Holidays

(previously published in *GRIT* magazine)

U NFORTUNATELY, holidays promote commercial hype, leading to wasteful consumerism. Each purchase we make directly affects the future of the Earth. Let's show love and compassion to the Earth during the holidays. Instead of buying flowers, buy a houseplant. Instead of buying a heart-shaped box of chocolates loaded with preservatives and artificial sweeteners, buy fairtrade organic chocolate. Instead of buying a card, make your own with recycled materials. Or instead of buying a gift, give an experience. For children, encourage them to make their own gifts from recycled materials.

Making your own gifts has many perks.

* Fulfill the intrinsic need to create. DIY gifting allows for a creative outlet; the process is fun and rewarding.
* Reduce your carbon footprint. Help eliminate the vicious waste cycle that is inevitable with the holiday season; reduce gas money and travel time by avoiding the shopping frenzy.
* Keep your sanity and dodge the crowds.
* Save money by using materials that you already have.

Follow these simple and creative ideas to make your own gifts for the special men, women and children in your life. Most of these gifts are so aesthetically pleasing that they don't even need to be wrapped. Just tie on a ribbon or attach a bow.

Eco-friendly Pillows

Use fabric, repurposed linens or painters' canvas (found in hardware stores). Cut two pieces of fabric the same size. Paint or stamp one of the pieces. Once the art has dried, face it art side down on the other piece. Sew the top three sides together using a sewing machine or needle and thread. Turn pillowcase

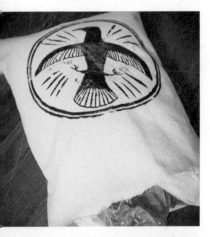

inside out. Stuff with recycled plastic grocery bags until you reach your desired shape. To complete, stitch up the bottom. These pillows are decorative and cannot be machine washed. Use a damp rag to spot clean.

Art Journal

Cut a piece of fabric roughly 16 inches by 9 inches. Cut three pieces of cardboard roughly 8 inches by 4 inches. Cut three pieces of heavy-duty fabric or leather roughly 8 inches by 4 inches. Sew the three pieces of cardboard evenly and with space in between onto the inside of the 16-by-9-inch piece of fabric. Sew the heavy-duty fabric or leather onto the cardboard to form pencil or marker holders. Sew a button on the front of the journal. Attach a piece of hemp to the button by tying several knots around the button. The journal can be closed by winding the hemp around the journal, then around the button.

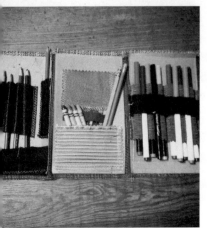

Cloth Journal

Use recycled cardboard, such as a used notebook cover. Grab a nice piece of fabric, an old piece of clothing or repurposed linen. Cut the fabric to the size of the cardboard or a little larger if you desire nice pleated and finished edges. Sew the fabric onto the cardboard with a sewing machine. Cut about 10 sheets of paper the size of your cardboard. Sew the paper onto the cardboard/fabric with one seam, right down the middle of the journal. Sew a button on the front. Attach a piece of hemp to the button by tying several knots around the button. The journal can be closed by winding the hemp around the journal, then around the button. Include a sharpened pencil or a nice pen with the gift.

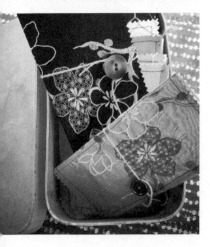

Easy Apron

Aprons can be made with any fabric such as old towels, t-shirts, sheets and linens. Add some art to the front, and voila, you have the perfect gift for the aspiring chef. Cut the fabric to the desired apron size. Fold the edges twice and sew to prevent fraying. On each side sew on straps that are at least 24 inches long.

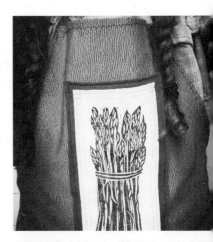

Birthday Calendars

Using just a few materials, this holiday gift is sure to please. These calendars are a timeless and non-technological method for remembering birthdays of friends and relatives.

Cut a piece of reclaimed wood (¼ inch thick) roughly 16 by 18 inches. Paint the wood if you choose. Hot glue pieces of ribbon, old straps or even strips of recycled cardboard onto the back of the wood. Write the word "Birthdays" and the months on the front of the wood. Write names and birthdays on tiny clothespins or fancy clips to hang on the ribbons for the appropriate months. Hammer two nails onto the top of the board and hang with a piece of wire or an old wire hanger.

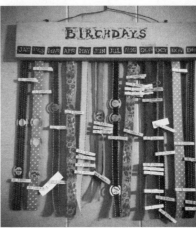

Simple Backpack

These simple backpacks are best made with a heavy duty fabric like corduroy or an old quilt. Since the backpack will most likely hold school supplies, cut the fabric large enough to accommodate them.

Step 1: Cut two rectangles (14 by 16 inches) of heavy duty fabric such as painters' canvas drop cloth, preferably used, an old cloth bag or repurposed quilt or blanket.

Step 2: Paint or decorate one piece of off-white muslin fabric (8 by 10 inches).

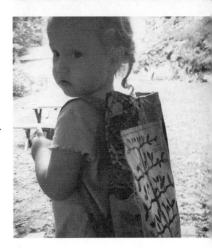

Step 3: Sew it to the side of the fabric that will show when the backpack is being worn.

Step 4: Hem the top edge of each of the rectangles (be sure the decorated side is facing the correct side).

Step 5: Add Velcro to each of the middle top inside sections of the rectangles, about 1 inch from the top hemmed edge. The Velcro will close the backpack once assembled.

Step 6: Place 2 rectangles together (design facing inward, Velcro facing outward)

Step 7: Sew the backpack together in a U shape, making sure the Velcro opening is facing up.

Step 8: Turn backpack inside out. Art/decorated rectangle should face out; Velcro should face in.

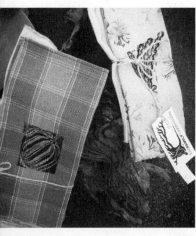

Step 9: Sew on straps of equal length (roughly 16 inches for children and 24 inches for adults). Use old belts, cloth bag handles or make your own by sewing together a 2-inch band of fabric. Make the straps thick enough to support the weight of the backpack, and sew them onto the top of the back-facing rectangle and the bottom of the backpack. Be sure not to sew the backpack together.

Cloth Napkins

Cut four equal pieces of old curtains or pillowcases and hem the edges. Paint or draw with a fabric marker on each napkin and gift as a set of four. Personalize individual napkins if you are making a family gift.

Unique Children's Stools

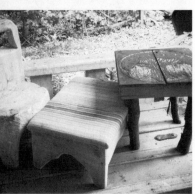

Get creative in the wood shop with these simple children's stool designs. For rustic stools, use a chainsaw with a newer chain to carve out a stump into the shape of a stool. For fancy stools, use fabric scraps or old linens to upholster tiny kids' furniture. For earthy stools, use sturdy branches as legs and reclaimed lumber for the top. Carve a design out or paint a pattern on top.

— Eric Stevens

Mason Jar Holder

Use screws to fasten hose clamps to a piece of reclaimed lumber. The hose clamps can be measured and tightened to hold Mason jars. Add hanging hardware to the back of the wood. Use to store pens and pencils, art supplies, dry goods, spices or anything your heart desires.

— Jason Crawford and Liz Meitus

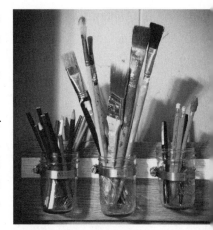

Elegant Mason Jar Vases

Create stunning vases using recycled glass jars with tape and paint. Use various widths of masking tape, painter's tape or scotch tape to make elegant patterns on glass jars. No need to buy several rolls of tape; simply cut the desired widths of masking tape. Paint or spray paint jars and remove tape once paint has dried.

— Jason Crawford and Liz Meitus

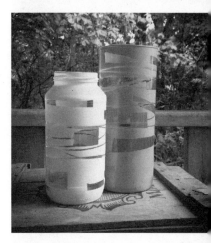

Rustic Woodland Art Vase

Create a beautiful piece of functional art that doubles as a rustic flower vase. Simply glue skinny branches of various lengths onto a jar with heavy-duty glue. This decorative jar could also hold art supplies, paint brushes or knitting needles, or could even be fashioned into a DIY lamp.

— Molly Hayden

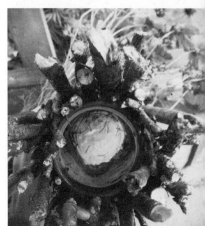

Jars of Fun

Fill Mason jars with toys for older children or use them as shelf decorations for younger children. Top with a plastic lid. Use your imagination as

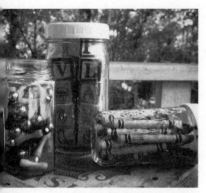

the possibilities are endless: marbles, arts and craft supplies, blocks, Legos, beads, jacks, bouncy balls, natural candies ... the list goes on!

Bow and Arrows and Fairy Wands

To make a bow and arrow, use a long pliable branch and tie a thin rope tightly to either end, bending the branch in an arch. Make arrows out of branches as well. Cut a piece of foam in a triangle and attach to the stick for the arrow.

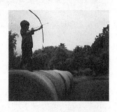

To make fairy wands, simply attach any decorative items you may have lying around to the end of a branch. Examples include artificial flowers, swirly q's, ribbons, bows, felt flowers and butterflies. Gift alone or paired with homemade cardboard fairy wings and a fabric scrap tutu.

Fort Kit

What's not to love about building a fort? Give a timeless gift that will inspire imaginative play! In a personalized pillowcase, combine repurposed household items such as old sheets, ropes, clothespins, twine, clamps and shoelaces. Add flashlights, batteries, playing cards and snacks for extra fun. Personalize for boys and girls of all ages.

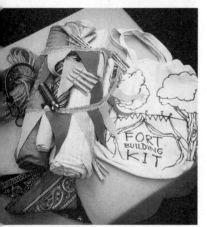

inspire

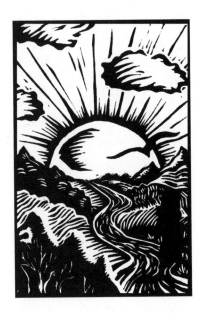

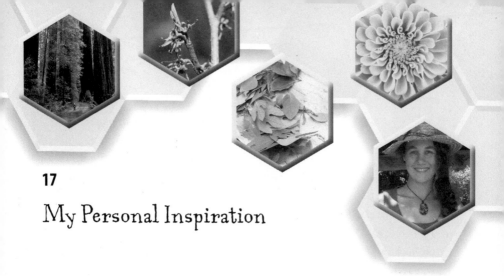

17

My Personal Inspiration

A FTER DEEPENING MY CONNECTION to food, to others and to the environment throughout the last decade, an overwhelming need to be a conduit in the global uprising came over me. Those in my generation including artists, poets, writers, growers, young homesteaders, do-it-yourselfers and greenhorns are experiencing this need to take part in global change. Historically, every generation has had its fair share of misfits, those who don't fit into the mass-approved social norm, those with progressive minds and lion hearts, those who are not afraid to fight the good fight and speak up for what they hold in their hearts to be true.

My Inspiration

After turning 30, I became uneasy about the status of my life at that time. I had wanted so badly to make my father proud and to accomplish lifelong goals, such as obtaining a degree in environmental science. But life had other plans for me. I had already started writing this book, but I was at a point of stillness with it, not knowing how to get it published or if it would even be worth it.

As I was sowing seeds in the high tunnel at La Vista on an early spring morning, I began to ask myself a series of questions.

> *How can I make my father proud?* I can do what I love, live with intent, do good for my family, inspire others.
> *What do I want to do with my life?* Finish my book, keep growing food, write and create art. Most importantly, I want to write.
> *What do you want to write about?* Sustainability, growing food and medicine, preparing seed-to-table recipes, nature, our relationship to the natural world, permaculture as a global solution.

Who can I write for? Mother Earth News, GRIT magazine, Permaculture magazine, The Healthy Planet, Feast Magazine.

As soon as I had these questions answered, I finished sowing seeds as quickly as I could and rushed home to start e-mailing pitches, proposals and my resume to all of these publications.

I was overwhelmed with joy and ambition! I had figured out exactly what I wanted to do! Within one hour of contacting JB Lester, publisher of *The Healthy Planet*, I received the go-ahead to write a six-page CSA guide for the St. Louis and the surrounding areas. I was beyond excited. Within three hours of submitting a proposal to the editors of *Mother Earth News* magazine, I received this response: "We are sorry we don't have any editorial openings at the moment, but we would love for you to blog for the magazine." I was elated. It was overwhelming to me that I essentially just manifested my dream scenario in less than five hours, just by asking myself a series of simple questions. I immediately started on my first blog post.

This was my very first post as a *Mother Earth News* blogger:

> *While* Mother Earth News *originated before I was born, it doesn't alter the notion that my life as I know it today is attributable to the inspiration I have found from the magazine throughout the years. I have been reading* Mother Earth News *for as long as I can remember. One of my earliest vivid childhood memories is sitting on my father's lap as a young girl reading* Mother Earth News *together in the 1980s and all throughout my childhood. He would read aloud while I studied the pictures of passive solar building, vegetable gardening, sheep shearing, building your own sugar shack and the beautiful array of topics which he read to me frequently.*
>
> *Those images, along with the camping trips in the mountains, the whitewater and canoeing excursions, and our family trip to Alaska, have been etched in the catacombs of my childhood memories and have sculpted the person I have grown to become.*
>
> *My father was a master carpenter and sourced a plethora of brilliant ideas for DIY building projects in his* Mother Earth News *magazines. My favorite was the swing set he built for my sister and me in California. While inspiration cannot be physically traced, I am certain that the streams of words I heard from my father's voice while my head was pressed against his heart and the smell of his*

morning coffee filled the air, inexorably educated me about the environmental issues which faced our society and inevitably moved me on a profound level to take action as an adult, all the while becoming educated and informed by reading Mother Earth News.

In 2000, my father was diagnosed with lung cancer. As a believer in natural medicine, I, along with my mother, convinced him to try Alternative medicine. I got a job at a local health food store in order to receive the 20% discount on organic foods and supplements. I worked in the juice bar and would bring him wheatgrass shots and fresh mixed vegetable juice after each shift. I remember reading articles in Mother Earth News on juicing and wheatgrass and learning their benefits on the systems of the body. My father's energy level significantly increased with each natural approach we took. He started seeing an acupuncturist, Dr. Sachs. My father showed tremendous results to Alternative treatments but to his demise, he did not give up smoking. The cancer then spread to his liver and his doctors strongly recommended chemotherapy and radiation. The stress of a culmination of exhausting treatments, living in the inner city, not being able to provide for his family, and unbearable pain eventually led to his deterioration. My father died in 2005. He left a beautiful legacy behind. He inspired many people in his lifetime.

One of the most important lessons I learned from him was that, "You don't need to have a lot of money in order to live a rich and fulfilled life. Beauty in the natural world is free and all around you, you just have to take the time to explore it." I am grateful for the insight and wisdom he bestowed upon me. The greatest tangible inheritance I received from my father was his collection of Mother Earth News magazines. Because of that collection of dusty magazines from three decades and my mother's support and encouragement to follow my dreams, I went on to become an herbalist and an Alternative Energy Practitioner and eventually a farmer. Everything I learned from reading Mother Earth News inspired me to make changes in my own life for a better planet. I have come to a place in my life where I love what I do. I work outside in a beautiful natural setting where native tall grasses blow in the wind, where migrating birds fly overhead by the thousands, where stillness and quiet reign over noise, where my children are close by and exposed to nature daily, and where my husband smiles, winks, and waves to me while passing by on the *bright orange battery powered Allis Chamers tractor on his way to cultivate a row of vibrant lettuce. Because of the impact my father made on me through his love for reading* Mother Earth News, *my dream has always been to write for the publication. I feel that inspiring others is a quintessential component to making the changes we wish to see in the world!*

Although I had been writing and journaling since I was 13, my writing career began by submitting proposals to magazines whose missions resonated with me on topics that I am truly passionate about. Anything is possible when you put your vision to action!

Miracles Happen Every Day

5-26-12: The day I met my brother... A day I will never forget.

"Miracles happen every day," is my mother's favorite saying. On May 26, I felt the truth of those words.

When my mother was 19, she gave up her son for adoption. He was born January 10, 1976. It was the most heart-wrenching day of her life and the hardest decision she ever made. She had a rough upbringing and was practically raising her younger brother and twin sisters. Having been through a series of traumatic events the year before she conceived, she was in no place mentally, emotionally or financially to raise a child of her own. She wanted a better life for her son, so she gave him up for adoption, hoping he would be raised by a loving and supportive family. As the years passed, my mother always wondered where he was and if he was being rocked to sleep, sung to, learning how to read and write and draw ... Not a day went by when he didn't cross her mind.

Years later, she met my father. They married and moved just outside of Denver, Colorado, where my sister and I were born at home. When I was five, we moved to California. After a year and a half, we returned to St. Louis and rented a tiny house in South City. They bought a rundown house on Compton, and my father, a carpenter, spent the next 13 years renovating it, one room at a time. I remember growing up in that house with sheets as walls for several years.

Every January 10, I would awake to the sound of my mother crying. I knew each year what ailed her. She wished she would have not made that life-changing decision and wanted more than anything to celebrate her son's birthday with him. As I matured, I understood more about what it meant to be adopted. I always had this gut feeling that I would meet my brother through my circle of friends. From the moment we got the internet at home in the late '90s, I started adding my mother's info to every online adoption registry that I could find. I searched for him on a regular basis but never with any luck.

In the spring of 2012, my mother got a call from a woman who asked her if she had given up a child for adoption. My mother's heart soared. She knew right away that the day had finally come. The woman was the mother of my brother's girlfriend. They had a daughter, and the three of them lived in Denver. He grew up in the very small town of Washington, MO, just miles from my parents' extended families. He went to school in Lawrence, KA, received a degree in architecture and was also a master craftsman, with skills he learned from his adoptive father.

It turns out that my brother's girlfriend and I share several circles of friends. My brother and and I enjoy a variety of similar interests, especially music and our love of art, gardening, craft beer and farm-fresh local foods. There is so much to this story ... enough to fill a book.

While my mother works on writing a book about the whole story, I will say this: meeting my brother and his family on that beautiful day, May 26, 2012, was one of the most profound experiences of my life. We all had been trembling with anticipation in the weeks leading up to the event. He welcomed us with open arms and spent a solid couple of hours with each of us individually. He shared a heartwarming slideshow of his life, adding sweet comments about each photograph. His eyes were bright and intense, and his smile was as beautiful as the mountains he traveled from. He was every-thing I had hoped for in a big brother: sweet, kind, patient, loyal, forgiving, honest, slightly sarcastic in an endearing kind of way and, above all, willing to love! I felt an instantaneous connection with my brother and his darling family. I cherished each story, smile and glance. I have so much respect and love for him. I am so impressed by his talents and abilities — they go beyond words.

I look forward to every form of communication from him. It makes my day when he sends me a text or shoots me an e-mail. I am so grateful to call myself his little sister, and I look forward to our many moons together in the future.

This anecdote plays a crucial role in my ability to grow as an individual and is a gentle reminder to keep hope alive, to love unconditionally and to find common ground.

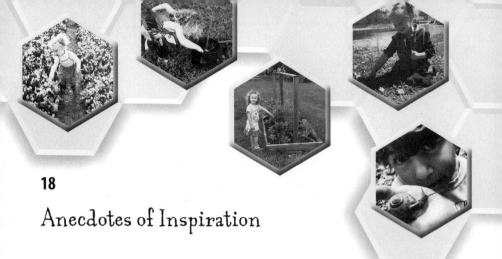

18

Anecdotes of Inspiration

THE WORLD IS VAST. Inspiration for the array of human capabilities, talents and expressions can be traced to every natural occurrence existing symbiotically in this ever-evolving ecosystem.

Music. Perhaps inspired by the melodies of birds, the rustling of leaves, the rhythms of nature, bullfrogs jumping into ponds, mating calls, the rain falling, the ebb and flow of the ocean ... Think of some of the most beautiful songs you've heard. Chances are the composers were inspired by nature in some way.

Art. Scenic landscapes brilliantly recreated by brushstrokes, nature artistically captured by photograph, still life, sculpture, pen and ink, pictograph, collage, etchings. Flowers recreated delicately on canvas with oil paint. Think about the art you love and how it was also inspired by nature.

Passionate artistic endeavors derive from our direct connection with nature. These endeavors feed our souls and bring about a jovial awakening within the very essence of our being, connecting our conscious selves viscerally with our deeper, soulful existence. They fuel our inner fire. They make our hairs stand on end. The desire to create fulfills us like nothing else does. It provides the pulse that moves us forward.

Inspiration is infinite. It is all around us. Our inspiration originates from nature: the patterns, the colors, the textures, the strength, the beauty, the continuous bounty, the endless breath, the symbiosis, the breathtaking scenery, the light, the sun, the darkness, the moon, the ocean, the stillness, the breeze, the horizon, the deserts, the canyons, the mountains, the foothills, the rivers, the streams, the lakes, the ponds, the rocks, the stones, the crystals, the rainbows, the caves, the vast universe, the cosmos, the stars, the storms, the earth, the sky and everything in between.

Inspiration is found on every street corner, in every office building, at every bus stop, in every school, in every church, in every supermarket, at every intersection and in every crack in the sidewalk from which thriving plants, against all odds, grow forth.

Inspiration is bounteous and infectious and too good not to be shared. Being inspired by others and inspiring through our own work is essential to making the changes we wish to see in the world! Inspiration can be found in a the song of a street musician, a single tree sapling in a clear-cut area, a family member surviving and overcoming an illness, a garden, a prairie. We just have to open our hearts to it, wherever it may be.

The Legacy of Jaime Hines

I met Jaime Hines in the spring of 2010 at La Vista Farm. She was the farmer at the Children's Discovery Garden. We became instant friends. I soon learned of her long battle with breast cancer. When we met, she was in remission and full of life. After being inspired by her enthusiasm despite having battled cancer, I decided to start hosting Luna Circles for her, to offer a place of healing and emotional release. The Luna Circles began with a small intimate group of Jaime's friends getting together with the equinox, solstice and select full moons. We would write our worries, fears and frustrations down on small pieces of paper and burn them in a fire. We would go around the circle, speaking of the pain, smudge each other with sage and then speak of our hopes, dreams and aspirations. Women have gathered since the dawn of humanity, forming a special bond that should be carried out generation after generation. Being in a safe and compassionate group of women is a form of emotional healing that all women need and deserve.

Jaime's cancer spread to her lymph nodes. Her jaw swelled to twice its normal size, but she remained optimistic, and the Luna Circles became more frequent. Her prognosis did not look good. Jaime lost hope. As a quick response to her devastation, I rounded up all of her close friends and acquaintances to make a friendship quilt for her. Each of us made a 12-by-12-inch square with a message for Jaime, and we stitched them all together to form a patchwork quilt, which we presented to her during a Luna Circle of over 40 women. She was so grateful to be a part of a loving and supportive group. At the next Luna Circle, on a chilly fall evening, she brought gifts for everyone. As she passed them out, a wave of emotion and genuine sadness came over all of us. As she handed each one our unique and personalized gifts, she expressed that she knew she wouldn't be here to celebrate any more of our birthdays. The tears were flowing. Our friend was dying. All of us drove home that night with heavy hearts and an overwhelming sense of gratitude for our own lives and families and all the tiny little miracles that happen every second of every day.

Jaime Hines spent years as the farmer at the Children's Discovery Garden. She instructed families on how to use sustainable practices to grow their own productive vegetable gardens. She taught workshops on square-foot and lasagna gardening, gave one-on-one instruction to families on a regular basis and was always doing nature crafts with kids and organizing successful fundraisers for the garden. She also co-taught Earthworms, a program that teaches children about gardening, science, plant identification and survival skills. Jaime was truly a selfless woman who dedicated her life to teaching others about sustainability.

Despite her less-than-desirable prognosis, Jaime shined and inspired others in ways that seem unimaginable by someone experiencing such turmoil mentally and physically in their own life. Her uphill battle with cancer caused many trials and tribulations, but miraculously, she had remained strong, radiant, loving and vibrant during her illness and has continued to inspire hundreds of children through her commitment and dedication to growing food for families. Knowing that people like Farmer Jaime have walked this Earth gives me hope for the future of humanity and of the environment. She was always innately passionate about teaching children and families how to be self-sufficient and how to make their own lives more wholesome through gardening. They have been working to preserve and protect the Earth for many years.

Jaime Hines left this world with the howling wind on a full moon just after midnight on March 16, 2014. Her legacy will be carried out by everyone dear to her. Sweet, loving, compassionate and adored by everyone who knew her, she will be forever heavy on their hearts and minds. Throughout her five-year battle with cancer, Jaime lived, loved and inspired more than most will do in a lifetime. She taught hundreds of children how to grow their own food and has inspired thousands of individuals throughout her journey. Her family and friends will continue her life's work through every future sustainable endeavor we attempt. She truly made this world a better place.

Legacy is defined as something that is received from or transmitted by a predecessor.

When it comes to the word "legacy," many of us might think of what we wish to leave behind once we are gone. After losing my dear friend Jaime, I reflected on the word, its true meaning and symbolism, and now have a newfound understanding. I wrote a blog post last summer titled "Children in the Garden" in honor of my vibrant friend, a remarkable woman and a wonderful mother. In many ways because of Jaime's legacy, I have dedicated the rest of my life to advocate for the Earth, to help protect the land and the living organisms, to create a living legacy through my own intrinsic moral obligation to the Earth as well as to ensure that her legacy will be carried on through seeds of hope.

Jaime inspired everyone around her to be a little more like her as they walk this journey on Earth. In an attempt to be more like the virtuous woman she was, I have prepared this mantra:

> Live out your legacy. Be the greatest you.
> Discover your passions and make them a part of your daily life.
> Tread a little lighter. Live with gratitude. Shine a little brighter.
> Let sorrow drift with the wind.
> Be steadfast with the seasons of change.
> Be optimistic, hopeful and joyful ... no matter the obstacle.
> Be kind and gentle to everyone.
> Love stronger.
> Be a catalyst for optimism.
> Plant more seeds, more flowers, more gardens, more trees.
> Be flexible and open to the winds of change.
> Honor the Earth and all of its components. Be genuine.
> Live out your legacy.

The Discovery Garden: A Model of Hope Through Gardening for Youth

Allowing children the space to discover the beauty and wonder of plants by tending to their own garden builds character, teaches responsibility, gives insight into the beauty of nature and connects them to their food source. The Children's Discovery Garden at La Vista Park in Godfrey, IL, is an excellent model for education and outreach through community gardening and is a beautiful example of how individuals from all walks of life can come together and fulfill a vision with love and support. Community Cultivators, an amazing group of Earth stewards, each play an integral role in its success and continued existence.

According to the Community Cultivators, interested community members and the Godfrey Parks District first met in 2001. After the board was formed and nonprofit status was awarded in 2002, the first group of children visited the garden in October. On Earth Day 2003, the official ribbon-cutting ceremony was held, and the garden obtained funding for its first paid employee.

The project goal is to "provide a gathering place for the children and their families to learn about the importance of organic gardening. They hope to promote the children's connection with the earth and the cycle of gardening. They also hope that people visiting the garden will have an increased appreciation of nature and how food is grown. The Discovery Garden is a place where the community and its children can come to participate in hands-on, creative outdoor activities while learning about food, community, volunteerism, and organic gardening."

Families pay a small annual fee for a specified plot to grow their own vegetable garden. Seeds and plants are donated by various organizations.

Solar Energy

One of the worst traits of humankind is our reliance on fossil fuels and the incessant depletion of nonrenewable resources. There are many alternatives, and yet the majority of the world still acquires energy using practices that are causing irreversible damage to the Earth, the people, the land, the air and the water. The exploitation of natural resources and reliance on coal-powered plants and nuclear energy plants will lead to a dismal future if solution-based renewable energy systems are not replaced as the norm.

The Power of One

Luckily, individuals like Aur Beck are shedding light on the easy transition to choosing renewable energy. My dear friend Aur "Da Energy Mon" Beck has been immersed in the growing field of renewable energy since he was a teenager. In 1990, at age 15, after independently researching solar energy, he moved into a 12-volt, battery-operated camper in his parents' driveway.

"Aur" translates as "light" or "to enlighten" in both Hebrew and Latin, a perfect name for a solar energy expert. According to Aur, "Reading profusely and consistently tinkering with renewable energy has been a continuous constant throughout my life. Never officially attending school left me time to do in-depth study, intern, view, and install renewable energy projects. Of course, working in one of the first United States passive solar schools helped."

Aur is the president, chief tech and coordinator of the Renewable Energy Install Network (Green Geek Squad) for Advanced Energy Solutions. Since

1999, he has been putting his knowledge to great use promoting, installing and educating on renewable energy.

Aur has made significant contributions to solar energy in recent years. He sheds his light in many ways:

* Founder and board member for both the Illinois Renewable Energy Association (illinoisrenew.org) and the Southern Illinois Center for a Sustainable Future
* Started Oil Addicts Anonymous International (IAmAnOilAddict.org)
* Hosts a weekly radio talk show called *Your Community Spirit* (Your CommunitySpirit.org)
* Helped AES Solar win the Missouri Schools Going Solar contract in 2005 and assisted with the sale and installation of 17 school systems
* Was a trained presenter for Al Gore's Climate Project in January 2007 (http://presenters.climaterealityproject.org/presenter/aur-beck_1006)
* Was invited to join the Midwest Solar Training Network (a Dept. of Energy program) (midwestsolartraining.org)

Aur grew up on a family farm in the heart of the Shawnee National Forest in an off-the-grid solar-electric-powered home, which makes it very easy to advocate for a life of simpler living, energy efficiency and renewable energy. He came up with and definitely lives by the Advanced Energy Solutions slogan, "We Empower YOU to Get Energized!"

I have been impressed with Aur's dedication to sustainable living and renewable energy since I first met him in 2000. One of his most notable accomplishments in the last few years was being invited by Neal Hinton, the dean of the School of Engineering and Information Technology of the Hocking College Energy Institute in Nelsonville, OH, to teach a semester of Solar PV Design and Installation. This is impressive because Aur has no formal college training; he is a living, breathing encyclopedia of all things solar. His ability to confidently teach at a college level is very inspiring. It not only encourages others to follow their dreams, but also offers a bit of insight into just how powerful it is to be passionate about what you do in life sans a degree.

At the Energy Institute, Aur inspired students by his "minds-on/hands-on" teaching methods. He tested their knowledge initially to try and fill in their education gaps, giving them useful and practical knowledge that had real-world applications. He was selected to teach due in part to the high failure rate and low test scores of students taking the NABCEP's (North American Board of Certified Energy Practitioners), entry-level program. He was able to change that into a high success rate. Renewable energy can reshape the future.

His company, Advanced Energy Solutions, offers:

* Solar- and wind-generated electricity
* Energy efficiency
* Utility-tied/net-metered or off-grid systems
* System design
* System and component sales
* Installation
* Onsite consulting and electrical load analysis
* Follow-up on technical assistance and service
* Training programs — designing and installing basic to advanced hands-on training labs

To learn more about Aur and his company, Advanced Energy Solutions Group, please visit his website aessolar.com. He also manages an off-grid living Facebook group, facebook.com/LivingOffGridReally.

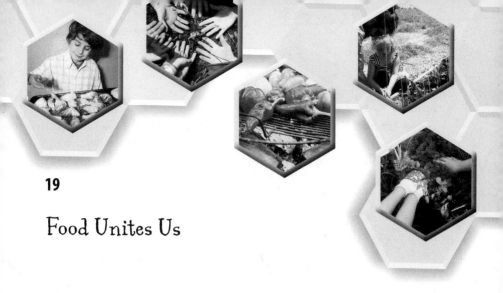

19

Food Unites Us

Joseph Simcox

J OSEPH SIMCOX, the "Botanical Explorer," is a seasoned ethnobotanist who has an intrinsic fascination with inherent wonders in nature. One of his keynote speeches, "Cavemen, Kings and Cannibals," which highlights how earlier civilizations revered food, addresses not only its nutritional components, but also the multitude of our historical relationships to food, including as power, a status symbol, a tool for influencing others, as well as its roles in extravagance, spirituality, ritual sacrifice and survival. One could spend hours listening to Joseph's stories of adventure and world travel. He speaks candidly of his trials in tracking down rare seeds, trials that were not limited to linguistic barriers!

Searching and asking questions is second nature for Joe, who was no ordinary child. He grew up in an ambiance where his parents fostered his inquisitive disposition from a very early age. His early life was immersed in science, exploration and books. Rather than play with toys, he found greater comfort exploring the world around him. He grew plants, searched for stones and cataloged seashells and insects. His passion for insects intensified his love of plants as he realized their mutualism. A budding botanist by the age of 12, he took pride in his impressive anthology of orchids, begonias and African violets. He lived vicariously through his specimens, imagining the astounding places they must have come from, resolving one day to see them in their native lands. Unbeknownst to him then, these collections would later define the very essence of his life's work — to ultimately increase awareness and appreciation of biodiversity of the plant kingdom by traveling the globe to identify, collect, grow and distribute seed from some of the rarest species known to man.

Joseph lives with gratitude and an overwhelming passion for the natural world and the symbiotic relationships that thrive in nature. His insatiable quest for tracking down plants and promoting languishing species keeps him searching by way of land, sea and sky. The great majority of plants are fascinating to him, but some shout out louder than others. All plants deserve respect, he says, and some more viscerally than others. Joe has been humbled by the sheer deadliness of some — he has been poisoned, blistered and scarred by their toxicities.

When not traveling, Joseph continues to study. He is enchanted by the myriad untold secrets veiled within nature and awed by the delicate beauty and intricacies within the anatomy of plants. Joseph contends that plants are our future, that we must learn how to create symbiotic relationships with them in order to live well on this planet. He invites us all to strengthen our affinity toward them, to take part in repopulating dwindling species, to plant native species to attract pollinators, to grow and save seeds from rare fruits and vegetables to reduce our reliance on large corporate farms and to spread the word to others on a daily basis. His fearless dedication to ecological preservation fuels his unwavering ambition.

Joseph, a steward of our Earth in the truest sense, dedicates his existence to bring awareness of the marvels of the plant world to as many people as possible. He hopes that by communicating his message he can incite a paradigm shift that changes the way we see and live with plants. Joseph holds on to the notion that "the world is a lot more resilient than we believe it to be." He believes that plants hold the keys to so many unanswered questions and that if we look to nature for solution-based models to follow, the world hunger issues would be few and far between. There are endless examples from his expeditions of food-producing plants that grow in environments ranging from barren sandy soil in hot deserts to frigid rocky mountaintops. The biodiversity at our disposal for eventual food production is so immense they obliterate the arguments touted by corporate industrialized agriculture for feeding the world.

Joseph's response to Monsanto's claim to feed the world is, "These institutions manifest a scenario that benefits the corporate and economic systems they helped create ... that has very little to do with real and legitimate strategies for creating a food-secure world." He speaks at conferences all over the world. His talks have taken him from the Asian Vegetable Research and Development Center in Shanshua, Taiwan, to the Central Tuber Crops Research Institute in Bhubaneswar, India, to the California Rare Fruit Growers annual Festival of Fruit conference, to the ECHO conference in Fort Myers, FL. He is a guest lecturer at universities, with this year's itinerary including Trinity College, Harvard University and the University of Hartford. Joseph is a leader of botanical expeditions that span the globe. His work represents history in the making as he changes the way the world perceives botanical diversity and how we stand to feed humanity in the not-so-distant future. Joseph's lively and exuberant presence captivates audiences wherever he goes. He speaks to people and conveys information equally well to children and professors. His passion is heartfelt and contagious.

When asked about his travels, he recalls years when he says he got off one plane only to get on another, logging millions of miles over the last several decades. He and his brother Patrick, also a "Botanical Explorer," have been fortunate enough to discover several species of plants that are still waiting to be named! They maintain a personal archive of almost 200,000 photos of edible plants from their travels, one that must rank among the largest self-acquired archives of its kind in the world.

Joseph is co-founder of The Rare Vegetable Seed Consortium, which has a collection of rare species of food-producing plants, one of the largest private collections in the world, with over 15,000 acquisitions. According to Joseph, "The Rare Vegetable Seed Consortium works to actively promote season-to-season cultivation, seed saving and sharing of its holdings of rare, non-GMO, heirloom genetic material." He also founded the Gardens Across America Project that works with gardeners in North America to promote seed preservation and encourage special seed grow-outs. Individuals or organizations can apply to be a host site for a few varieties of rare seeds, which involves growing, harvesting and saving the seed, and returning half of the saved seeds to Joseph and his team for further promotion.

On Joseph's team are his colleague Irina Stoenescu, his brother Patrick, his daughter Alicia, his brother-in-law Jason Piper, his sister Susan, young filmmaker Anthony Rodriguez and communications liaison Christine Chiu.

His latest expedition to the Amazon was in search of rare fruits and vegetables native to the Peruvian rainforest. Filmed by Anthony, it will be edited and condensed into several short films and a 45- to 60-minute documentary about food plant diversity in the Amazon.

Joseph's work is also featured in *Seed: The Untold Story*, released in early 2016.

When asked to name his favorite plants from various world expeditions, Joseph says that it is a tough question to answer. When I had the opportunity to pin him down on this, he shared some of the following:

- *Amorphophallus*, in Borneo
- *Hippophae rhamnoides*, berries found in the Russian taiga

- *Gnetum africanum*, a vining plant with medicinal and edible properties, found in Africa and farmed in Cameroon
- *Oromo dinich*, a mint family tuber-bearer in Ethiopia
- *Opuntia basilaris*, a spring-flowering cactus in the Mohave Desert
- *Lewisia* species, bitterroot, in the northwestern mountain states
- *Lomatium latilobum*, desert parsley, in Moab
- *Oplopanax horridus*, Devil's club, in the Pacific Northwest
- *Pholisma sonorae*, a rare perennial herb called sandfood, in the Sonoran Desert
- *Monodora myristica*, a fruit tree in Cameroon
- *Coccinia abyssinica*, a nutritious tuber-bearing plant in the cucumber family in Ethiopia
- *Solanum gilo*, a scarlet eggplant from Brazil
- *Cucumis humifructus*, the rare aardvark pumpkin, which grows underground, one of the only plants with subterranean fruits in southern Africa
- *Cucumis metuliferus*, the African horned cucumber, found in the Kalahari Desert
- *Tylosema esculetum*, the Maramba bean, found in the Kalahari Desert
- *Acanthosicyos horridus*, the nara melon, only found in Namibia
- *Telfaria pedata*, the oysternut, found in Africa
- *Pandanus conoideus*, red fruit found in south-central New Guinea
- *Pandanus tectorius*, Nicobar breadfruit, found in tropical coastal regions
- *Dolichos fangitsa*, an edible root that tastes like a watermelon, found in Madagascar
- *Prainea limpato*, a gorgeous edible tart and sweet fruit, found in Malaysia, Borneo and New Guinea
- *Dendroseris litoralis*, the cabbage tree, a perennial flower in the Asteraceae family that has been revived from near-extinction. It is native to the Juan Fernandez Islands near Chile.
- *Willughbeia elmerii*, a rare fruit found in the jungles of Borneo
- *Diospyros texana*, a black persimmon tree native to Texas and the southwestern United States
- *Peniocereus greggii*, a cactus native to the southwestern United States that has a root weighing more than 80 pounds. These cactuses only bloom for one night each year, typically in June or July.

⊛ *Cynomorium coccineum*, a parasitic flowering plant that has been used historically for its medicinal benefits

His present holy grail, one he has spent the last decade searching for and yearns to track down, is Hydnora africana with ripe fruit. This plant lacks chlorophyll, does not perform photosynthesis and takes upwards of two years for its fruit to ripen. The fruit grows underground. Finding Hydnora africana with ripe fruit would allow him to add yet another marvel to his "have eaten it" life list, one that already numbers in the thousands. If only for what this man can tell us about food plants, Joseph is an individual we can all listen to with fascination, because he knows it — food — like few of us ever will.

Food Unites Us

Food is the common thread weaving humanity together and is vital to our sustenance. Our waking hours are determined by our next meals; we gather to eat; sharing a meal is the most universal form of socialization. Everything in this world (every idea, dream and vision) is powered by the energy and nutrients we receive from our food. Cultures are defined by the foods they have grown and eaten since the dawn of humanity. Food has built the foundation of individuals, cities, nations and countries. Historically, individuals took part in daily tribal endeavors to grow their very basic food needs. Settlers and nomads alike built their lives around the food they could grow or forage in the wild.

The local foods movement is no new endeavor. It began over one million years ago with the first hunter-gatherers eating only what they could find in a 100-mile radius. The movement peaked during the victory garden days in the early 1900s when canning and preserving fruits and vegetables was a benchmark enterprise. Unfortunately, how humans revere their food sources has dramatically declined in the last 60 years.

Daniel Quinn, author of the *Ishmael* series, pinpointed the demise of civilization to growing food as a commodity, growing food for profit, which prompted the destructive practice of monoculture globally. This modern exploitation of sustainable archaic agrarian lifestyle changed the world and caused a massive disconnect of humans from their food. The local foods movement took a long hiatus during the Industrial Revolution and stayed in the background with the growth of grocery store chains in the 1950s. It has made a significant comeback in the last few years. Conscious eating seems to be the modern-day trend, and individuals worldwide are realizing again the importance of food: where it comes from and how it is grown. The rise of food awareness is paramount to our growth as a healthy, sustainable community. Supporting local food systems reduces our carbon footprint and circulates funds back into the local economy.

Grow Create Inspire examines how growing food through various permaculture-inspired techniques can help to create a momentum of inspiration to heal the Earth and change the future. I examine how permaculture is the one solution to all of the problems surrounding food. Permaculture is really at the heart of all solutions to the environmental, social and political issues facing the world today. It gives hope to humanity. Permaculture in action is so beautiful to witness and be a part of.

Food is Free Project

(originally published in *Permaculture* magazine)

One of the most inspiring permaculture stories I have heard from the food movement is the story that began in January 2012 with one seed, planted by one individual, that grew so beautifully into the Food is Free Project. Throughout history, creative, solution-based ideas tend to repeat themselves as elders pass down knowledge to the next generation. Inspiration is cyclical and a cog for motivation. The Food is Free Project was founded by John VanDeusen Edwards, whose grandfather, Earle Edwards, was a conscientious objector to World War II and planted apple trees instead. John believes we can live in a world beyond war, a world where we can connect with each other through our food. He was reinspired after reading a gardening book that stated, "As gardeners, we all have an obligation to share this knowledge about growing food for ourselves and others and to keep the tradition of gardening alive." John, a former insurance salesman, believes strongly that people from all walks of life are capable of taking steps toward a more sustainable world by simply starting in their own front yard with a garden. He couldn't be more elated to have left the chaotic world of nine-to-five hustle and bustle, going from chasing money to chasing dreams. He is a wonderful example of how being rich is not about the numbers on our bank statements, but the value of our lives and the beautiful ways in which we can be fulfilled: mind, body and spirit. He now focuses all of his time and energy on the Food is Free Project.

> I truly believe that planting a garden is a revolutionary act that is coming from a place of love.
>
> — John VanDeusen Edwards

John was inspired in 2012 after hearing about wicking bed gardens, a low-maintenance raised bed idea that could be made with basic affordable materials. He created his first wicking bed garden in his own front yard out of reclaimed pallets, political signs, a weed barrier, pea gravel, a plastic tarp, soil, an L-shaped PVC pipe and soil. After planting it, he placed a simple sign nearby, "Food is Free." This single act inspired a food revolution in Austin, TX. John got so much positive feedback about his front-yard free garden, he decided to become a catalyst of positive change for his neighborhood. He knocked on the doors of every house on his block and handed each neighbor a flyer that said, "The first 10 people who respond to this flyer will receive a free raised bed garden installed in their front yard." Talking to neighbors has become a lost art, and the fact that John took this first leap is remarkable. He went from not knowing any of his neighbors in the two years he had lived there, to knowing them all within a few days.

The responses were overwhelming, and within a couple of weeks, he, his friends and about 50 volunteers created ten wicking beds in the front yards along Joe Sayers Avenue. Within just one month, the Food is Free Project was born, and they had built 19 wicking beds on their street using materials sourced locally for free or donated. Nineteen out of 30 houses on Joe Sayers Avenue now have front yard free gardens, thanks to John and the dedicated friends of the Food is Free Project. Their neighborhood has come to life and has become a safer and friendlier place to live.

The Food is Free Project is now a 501c3 nonprofit organization whose mission is:

> to grow community and food, while helping gain independence from a broken agricultural system. The Food is Free Project is a community building and gardening movement which aims to inspire others to line their neighborhood street with front yard community gardens which provide free harvests to anyone.

According to John,

> The gardens are built and offered for free using salvaged resources that would otherwise be headed to the landfill. By using drought-tolerant, wicking bed gardens, these low-maintenance gardens only need to be watered every 2 to 4 weeks. This simple tool introduces people to a very easy method of growing organic food with very little work. A wide variety of vegetables

along the block promote neighbors to interact and connect, strengthening our communities while empowering them to grow their own food.

Since its inception, the Food is Free Project has gone global; not only has it received over 80,000 followers via social media in just two years, but it has truly sparked a movement, evoking a visceral uplifting emotion of hope in humanity in individuals worldwide, including myself. John receives e-mails daily from individuals, groups and organizations around the globe showing their support for his vision. Daily, hundreds from each continent post photographs of their own "food is free" projects sparked by John's simple yet brilliant idea. This movement goes beyond the local foods movement. It breaks down barriers and builds bridges. It unifies people from every race, creed and color. It strengthens the bond we all share to our food. The Food is Free Project is truly a game changer.

By 2013, John and his partner, Stacey Volland, turned their yard into a fully functioning half-acre urban farm and education center. Their backyard chickens provide fresh eggs for their intentional community. At their outdoor kitchen, they teach nutrition, food preparation and preservation classes. They are now a host site for gardening, permaculture, hugelkultur and beekeeping workshops as well as a variety of other sustainability-focused workshops. They have become a drop-off location for pallets, political signs, recycled buckets, gardening supplies, seeds and plants. They started a community composting program, using compost that people drop off to make soil to share with neighbors. Their goal is to keep expanding to integrate youth programs, school field trips and other outdoor learning-based programs. John's good friends, Trystan Puckhaber and John Van Lowe, have been in it with him since the beginning, each bringing a creative and innovative flair to the project.

John is full of gratitude for being surrounded and supported by such an amazing community. He believes the Food is Free Project has the potential to make neighborhoods safer and foster healthy, happy communities. The use of political signs brings a brilliant and positive approach to uniting both the Democratic and Republican parties to form the "Garden Party." Seeing people from all walks of life coming together in the collective vision of building a more sustainable and practical food system is one of John's favorite aspects of the project. Thriving together instead of surviving alone helps to strengthen the bond that unites us human to human and helps us to build resiliency.

Open the lines of communication within your own community. Call political organizations and ask them for signs; call the local parks and recreation office to ask for soil donations. Ask local businesses if they will donate pallets. John encourages everyone to mention the "Food is Free Project" name when soliciting donations. Much of his experience in asking for donations has been positive, and he finds that businesses are eager to become involved.

Wicking Bed Garden

The wicking bed garden, essentially a handmade aquifer inside of a raised bed, is typically 4 feet by 4 feet when made from pallets.

Materials (90 percent donated or sourced locally for free):

- 2 pallets (heat-treated): Acquired free from local businesses who would otherwise pay to have them picked up
- Recycled political signs: Contact local campaign offices, which typically have a surplus that they are more than willing to donate.
- Scrap wood: Ask your neighbors or scour construction sites.
- Recycled crushed tumbled glass: Acquired from local landfills or recycling centers. Resource-recovery facilities often give tumbled glass for free. Use pea gravel or river rock as alternative, often acquired for free at construction sites.
- 10 to 12 inches of soil: Acquired for free at most city parks
- Tarp or plastic liner: Can be found for as little as 2 dollars

Visit foodisfreeproject.org/resources for a basic tutorial on how to build your own wicking bed garden.

John recently attended the March Against Monsanto in the US, where he gave away thousands of seedlings and planted hundreds of vegetable transplants into public planters. He stood on the steps of the Texas state capitol and spoke these words:

> It's time we take back our food and meet our neighbors. Invite your friends to join the mission. Transform your own neighborhood by planting a community garden in your front yard. By getting creative and working together with others, we can build a new food system from the ground up which not only localizes our food needs, but also brings our vibrant communities together in a safe and transformative way. This new way we start looking at food has the power to withstand the test of time.

The Food is Free Project is an open source movement. Feel free to use the name "Food is Free Project" to spark inspiration in your own corner of the world and in your own community. The project leaders are eager to hear about your alternatives to gathering resources and building wicking bed gardens. John welcomes everyone to post photographs or memes (#foodisfree) of your endeavors to the Food is Free Project Facebook page. Help them reach one million likes (facebook.com/foodisfree)! Visit www.foodisfreeproject.org to get inspired!

Spotlight on Earth Stewardship: Jere Gettle, Founder of Baker Creek Heirloom Seeds

On several occasions, we were artisan vendors at Baker Creek Heritage Festivals. In order to be a vendor, you are required to dress in "old-timey attire," which we happily did and enjoyed every second of it. Being in Bakersville Pioneer Village is like stepping back in time. The wide array of attractions include a mercantile store, an "apothecary shoppe," an enormous chicken coop with beautiful heritage breeds, stunning gardens, a metal smith exhibit and even the Bakersville Opry, complete with straw bale seating. It is truly a gardener's paradise. Like so many other patrons of Baker Creek, Jere and his wife, Emilee, have inspired my husband and me as farmers, parents, dreamers, artists and stewards of the Earth. They are a beautiful example of how one can manifest their own reality by transforming an idea into a dream, a dream into a vision and that vision into reality through hard work and perseverance, as well as unconditional support and encouragement from loved ones. Keep dreaming!

I had the opportunity to interview Jere for my blog with *Mother Earth News*. I've reproduced our conversation here, for it contains many lessons that I have kept with me to this day.

Jere Gettle always had a passion for growing things, and at age three, he planted his first garden. From early age, he wanted to be involved in the seed industry. So at the age of 17, he printed the first small Baker Creek Heirloom Seed catalog in 1998. The company has grown to offer 1,450 varieties of vegetables, flowers and herbs — the largest selection of heirloom varieties in the US.

Q: *What inspired you to be a steward of the Earth?*

Being in the garden as a child with parents and grandparents. Planting a tiny seed and watching it transform into the amazing diversity of fruits and vegetables. Being at eye-level with insects and seeing the part they play in our larger world. Watching the genetics of plants unfold right in front of my eyes.

Q: *What major obstacles have gotten in your way?*

Lots and lots of smaller hassles have worked together to create obstacles. Shortage of time is always a factor — there never seems to be enough time. Insect pests are always obstacles to anyone trying to grow things organically. Genetic engineering and cross-contamination mean that we have to spend time and money testing our seeds. We not only lose the immediate crops that have been contaminated, but are in danger of losing whole varieties themselves. Regulations on the movement of seeds create obstacles.

Q: *To you, what are the five most pressing environmental issues?*

1) Genetic engineering, because it threatens the whole history of farming and the future of food we eat. Genetic engineering even has the ability to threaten nature itself.

2) Increased application of pesticides, which is due in part to genetic engineering

3) Big-box stores

4) Factory farms, due to their impact on local communities and the massive runoff from them that pollutes our water systems

5) Mass transportation of food over long distances. Not only the carbon footprint created by the fuels themselves being used to transport food, but the added chemicals, waxes, gases, etc. that are used to make food travel well

Q: *What would be your five solutions to those issues?*

1) Label GMOs so people would have a choice to know what they are eating. Better yet, ban GMOs.

2) A decrease in genetically engineered crops would naturally lead to a decrease in pesticides. I would also increase education and make people aware of the dangers of GMOs so more people would be less likely to use pesticides if they knew the dangers.

3) The first step would be to educate people to the advantages of shopping locally. Have them get to know and trust the producers of their food. Another solution would be to take away the tax incentives and

monetary advantages that big-box stores and corporations are given over local businesses.

4) Take away the massive government subsidies given to factory farms, make them adhere to humane practices, limit the use of chemicals and antibiotics, as well as regulate runoff.

5) Encourage people to eat locally and grow their own food. Educate people about the advantages of eating foods that have been grown locally.

Q: What steps are you taking personally to contribute to a brighter future for the planet? On a local, national and global level?

I founded Baker Creek Heirloom Seeds to help preserve heritage seeds. I try to buy local and support local endeavors. I educate people about our historic food systems. I feel it is important that we all work towards establishing and supporting more localized food systems, localized markets and localized governments.

Q: What are your current projects?

At Baker Creek Heirloom Seeds' Petaluma Seed Bank, we are always constantly searching for new varieties of seeds to trial. We have a major restoration project underway at Comstock, Ferre & Co. that we purchased a few years ago in Wethersfield, CT. We are in the process of creating a food-related nonprofit organization. We are currently planning our third annual National Heirloom Exposition, a huge pure food event in northern California.

Read more about their current projects online at rareseeds.com.

Inspiration on the World Wide Web

Over Grow the System is an online nexus for sustainability activism, founded by Syd Woodward, a West Coast-based artist, photographer, filmmaker and blogger. His work is committed to deepening our relationships with and roles in building a truly resilient future. I have seen his work directly inspire individuals around the globe to start food revolutions in their own communities.

According to Woodward, the vision for Over Grow the System is to "create an effective and compelling platform that can empower and activate people across social spectrums, while also addressing the real issues and challenges that the world faces today. A platform that can inspire people to reclaim their freedom and their power from the cultural mechanisms of control and complacency in order to live more in balance with the cycles and systems of the natural world."

Their values:

* Live simply: Cultivate a consciousness shift to see that doing with less actually improves quality of life rather than compromises it.
* Right livelihood: Work should be in service to the natural world (that includes humans).
* Community: Work should empower and build community.
* Inspired: Live a life that is inspired and in turn inspire others.
* Action: Take action in the world and empower others to do the same.

Their projects include Free Range Child, Sea to Seed, Women Who Farm and Stories from a Fertile Earth.

Syd and his partner, Hemmie, continue to empower and inspire others to be resilient through gardening and to educate their communities about Earth stewardship, self-sufficiency and ecological awareness.

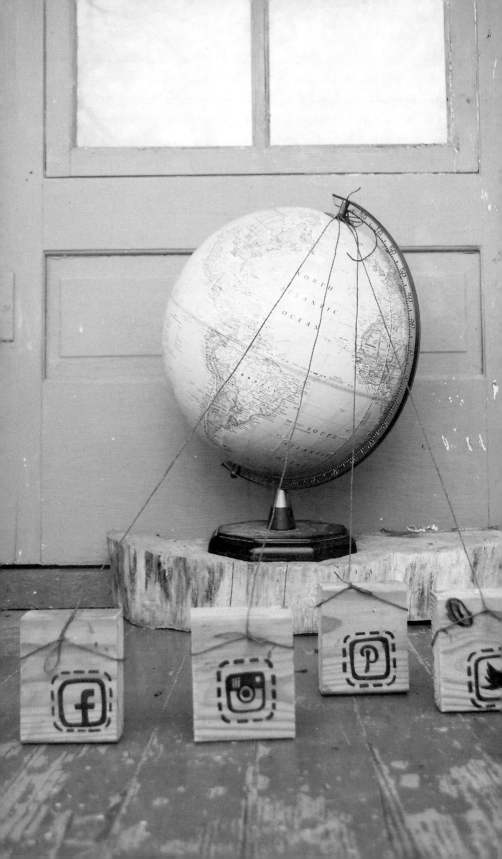

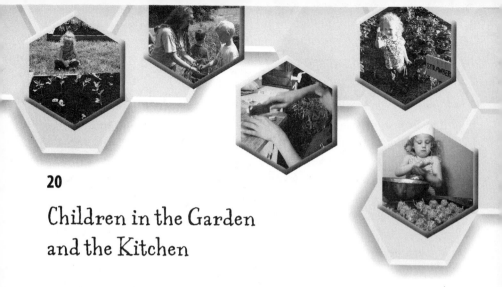

20

Children in the Garden and the Kitchen

WHEN A CHILD is allowed the opportunity of solo exploration among fields of green, a cognitive awakening occurs. A visceral chord is struck. The intrinsic survival instincts kick in. The mind, body and spirit unite, guiding the child to get back to the essence of nature. The child hears the sounds of crickets, birds, leaves rustling, the call of the wind. Their eyes open wide to all the wonders of nature. Their eyes dance across the horizon, witnessing the colors, textures, patterns, shapes and lines come to life. They notice the tiny beautiful intricacies of nature. They get down, knees pressed to earth and look at the tiny world that is thriving beneath their feet. The smell of the earth is rich and familiar. They taste the flavors of the earth: the sweetness of berries, the bitter dandelion greens, the crisp fresh food from their gardens and the salty sweat which drips from their cheek as the sun crosses the skyline. They become in tune with the rhythms, the seasons, the cycles of the natural world.

Children thrive when they are given great responsibility. To tend to the land and to care for a garden instills in them something that stays with them their entire lives. Knowing how to grow food is so vital to the future of humanity. All children should be given this beautiful opportunity.

Our son was born with severe medical complications. He has been virtually free of medical complications for many years now, and I believe a large portion of the phenomenon is because of his healthy diet and natural herbal remedies. Since he has healed from major complications, I became an herbalist and have been treating our children with mild medicinal herbs for each ailment whenever possible.

I use culinary herb tea for cold and flu symptoms, mullein and garlic oil for earaches, ginger peppermint tea when there are bellyaches ...

I find that the best way to get our kids to take herbs is to steep a tea, sweeten with honey and then pour into popsicle molds and freeze for them to enjoy as soothing cool treats.

I made our son's baby food by just taking what I made for us and blending it in the food processor. He learned to eat healthy food with lots of flavor right from the start. Of course, I slowly introduced the flavor. I began with just simple foods such as mashed sweet potato, avocado, squash or banana, but slowly added what was on our menu. We are very grateful for his positive attitude toward healthy food. We did the same process with our daughter with equally great results.

Our daughter was born into the beautiful world of sustainable farming. When Iris was just a week old, we photographed her in a basket of produce we had harvested that morning. For the first ten months of her life, she survived solely on breast milk loaded with concentrated nutrients from the homegrown produce I ate daily, most of which I ate raw directly in the field. You can imagine the nutrition of produce eaten within minutes of harvest. When Iris was ready for solid food, we pureed veggies from the garden. Her favorites were butternut squash and sweet potatoes. She learned how to pick peas before she could walk. She has thrived on the garden's nutritious bounty.

At four, our daughter has more knowledge than I did at age 16. She knows how to grow, how to weed, how to harvest and how to cook.

She runs the fields barefoot. She sings to the crops and dances for the plants. She is curious and brave, intelligent and wise, sweet and compassionate, loving and nurturing. She is four, but she is wise like the sages. She teaches me so much about life and love and healing.

She knows about herbal medicine. A budding herbalist, she collects plantain leaves when her friends get stung or bitten. She collects chickweed, violets, dandelion greens and flowers in the spring for salads. She helps us plant thousands of seeds in the high tunnel. In the summer, she weeds and waters the crops with us. She picks purslane and lamb's quarters and feeds it to us while we work. She helps carry cabbage down 100-foot rows. She harvests garlic with us and peels it. In the autumn, she harvests the bounty with us. She picks peppers (100 peppers in ten minutes). She loves pulling garnet beets and vibrant carrots from the earth. She arranges the produce artfully in produce baskets to photograph. In the winter, she draws pictures of us (her family) in the fields. She designs gardens and speaks of another harvest.

Food is an essential and beautiful part of our lives. It nourishes our bodies, gives us energy and strength and is incredibly delicious. And, of course, it plays such an integral role in our health. It is especially important for children to establish healthy eating habits at a young age. As parents, we are able to set good examples by eating healthy and by serving healthy foods. For most parents, it is a challenge to get their children to eat healthy foods. It takes a little time and creativity to get your kids hooked on healthy eating habits, but in the end, it certainly is worth it.

Encourage your child to develop a sophisticated palate and an appetite for healthy foods. Let them create art on their plates. Some of Iris and Cay's favorites are goat cheese, smoked salmon, massaged kale salad, broccoli and avocados. They are also very fond of green smoothies — fruit smoothies blended with kale and spinach or lettuce greens and spirulina. They prefer dark chocolate over processed candy loaded with sugar any day of the week. Some may disagree, but the method we used from the time they started eating was simply that they were required to eat everything that we served them. If they didn't like something, they had to learn to like it because first, it is good for them and second, that is what's for dinner.

The beginning of each new school year presents the perfect opportunity to get back into healthy routines. Summer is so busy, and we often build up a few less than desirable habits such as staying up late, sleeping in, avoiding structure and making unhealthy food choices. Because children focus and function better when they eat well-balanced meals, it is very important to make healthy food choices a part of their daily routine. Here are some ideas to provide some enjoyable structure and learning opportunities for your children.

Visit a farm. This is an excellent opportunity for children and their parents to spend some time feeling the earth beneath their feet, the wind in their hair and the sun on their backs as they pick nature's bounty and get in touch with the Earth that provides for us. One great way to experience the you-pick areas of a farm with children is to make it into a picnic. Spread a blanket under a shade tree while at the farm and have a picnic of fresh field-picked veggies.

Grow a garden together. Let them pick out the seeds, pick the spot where the garden will grow and give them the responsibility of watering and weeding. Witnessing the seed-to-table process gives children a greater understanding of where their food comes from.

Let your child use knives (you may be waiting for a line that reads "just kidding," but I am actually serious). They feel like a ninja, and if they are allowed to cut their own veggies and fruits, they are more likely to eat veggies and fruits. My kids go to a Montessori school. When my son was five, I came to pick him up early one afternoon during his first month there. When I got to the classroom, I saw him in the tiny play kitchen area using what looked like a giant meat cleaver to cut an apple. I frantically rushed over to him and said, "Buddy, no no no, this is for grown-ups." The teacher came running over and said, "Mrs. Stevens, this is the task he is working on right now. This is the practical life area of the classroom." I felt both embarrassed and slightly disturbed. When we came home that night, I gave him a cutting board, some celery and peppers, and a mini-meat cleaver. He did in fact chop those veggies like a ninja. From that moment on, I have become quite comfortable letting him use knives to help chop vegetables. Now nine, he has helped make many delicious soups. Teaching proper safety is key.

Let them play with their food! To help encourage them to try new things, make veggie funny faces, veggie superheroes and action figures (carrot bodies, peeled squash capes, parsley hair) and veggie and fruit portraits.

Buy healthy food or let them choose it. Instead of heading straight for the chips and cookies, take them to the produce section first to choose their favorite fruits and veggies. Skip the sugary snacks. Instead of cookies, send dark chocolate. Instead of fruit snacks, send real fruit. Instead of luncheon meat, send avocado sandwiches. Instead of junk food, send veggie sticks and dip.

Let them help plan meals. Let them browse through your cookbooks and choose their favorites. Let them help with prep!

If you follow any one of these suggestions, you will find that kids actually do like vegetables! They just need to be given the chance to explore the dizzying array of flavors and textures so they can learn to identify their tastes and distastes.

A Sprouting Experiment

My husband and I are continually looking for opportunities to teach our children about plants. I was showing my son all of the different seedlings in the high tunnel last spring, actively thinning trays while letting him sample micro-greens, including broccoli rabe, cauliflower, cabbage and even tiny shoots of scallions and herbs. He was very interested in the different colors and flavors of the plants. He was eating the baby green sprouts faster than I could thin them. My husband said something to me last year that stuck with me after I had expressed my fear of our son becoming detached from nature as technology entered his life at such a rapid rate. He said, "We know now that if he shows excitement about plants or nature that we drop everything and embrace his interest." That is our motto now, and we never stray from that. So when I asked him if he wanted to do a sprouting experiment so that he and his sister could learn more about plants and then eat the micro-greens as they grow, his eyes lit up.

He was enthusiastic about another process of growing his own food. He decided that our theme would be, "Which will sprout first?" He liked the idea of a "sprouting race." We gathered our supplies and set up the experiment at our kitchen table. As I made dinner, he wrote out the procedure, the hypothesis and the variables. He even asked if we could make a video. So we did. After thumbing through our sprouting seeds, he selected five different kinds of seeds to sprout: broccoli, sunflower, alfalfa, cauliflower and cabbage. His hypothesis was that broccoli would sprout first. He filled the tray with soil, poked holes in each cell, wrote his labels, planted his seeds, covered them with soil and gave them a gentle drink. He recited the elements that plants need to grow. He was so excited about the opportunity to eat micro-greens anytime he wanted. While broccoli did not win the race, this did not hinder his enthusiasm toward the experiment. Variations of this experiment could include observing plant growth during a full moon, placing the same potted seeds in different windows around the house, duplicating the process but adding a clear plastic lid and any other creative idea that the little sprout comes up with.

So if you give a boy a seed, he will plant it, watch it grow, possibly draw it, be amazed by it and more than likely eat the food that it produces. Watch their creativity sprout!

Back-to-Nature Lesson Plan for Kids

I regularly teach a children's summer camp program called Back to Nature at the nearby Montessori school. The daily curriculum journal can be used as a resource for nature-based activities and lessons for children. It can be a one-week lesson or can be easily expanded into a continuous lesson plan.

Day One. We started the morning with several questions:

1) Why do we need the Earth?
2) What is an Earth steward? Why is it important to be a steward of the Earth?
3) What is nature? Are we a part of nature?
4) Why do we need nature?

After each child had a turn to answer the questions, they created name tags using recycled materials. I asked them to draw a plant, animal or insect on their name tag.

We then went outside for an introduction to the concept of the web of life. For this I used a ball of yarn. The plant, animal or insect drawn on each name tag represented living components in the food chain of the web of life. I held the end of the yarn and introduced myself, showing them that I drew a dandelion plant on my name tag. I asked the class to think about which animal on their name tags would possibly eat a dandelion. After glancing around the circle, all the children shouted out, "a rabbit." Once the boy with the rabbit on his name tag agreed, I threw him the ball of yarn, while still gripping on to the end. We created a food web by determining, as a group, who eats what. By the end, the children knew the names of the other plants and animals and whether they were a predator or prey. Each held onto the strand of yarn weaved together by the interrelationships between plants and animals.

We then trekked out to the garden that we planted during last year's summer camp garden class. We hand-pulled the crabgrass that was growing against the stones and used a broad fork and a garden hoe to turn under the soil. I gave a tutorial about starting your very own garden with just a little space and a few simple tools. After demonstrating how to use each tool efficiently, I gave everyone a few minutes with each tool in the ten-foot garden plot. I asked one student to set his stopwatch for 20 minutes. We had the soil turned under in 16 minutes. We went in for a refreshing glass of fennel and basil-infused water.

We talked about the wonders of the world and the importance of protecting the last remaining wild areas. We discussed deforestation, strip mining and mountaintop removal, as well as air and water pollution. I gave the children several examples of how they can help our environment by reducing their carbon footprint and by living by the daily principles of the three R's. I showed them a brilliant documentary, *The Story of Stuff*.

We then went for a nature walk, and each child picked a dozen objects from nature. Back in the classroom, we identified a few from each child's collection, and they made nature collages. For a snack, I brought a large bowl of peas that we grew at La Vista Farm.

Day Two. We started the morning with a meditation. We discussed the importance of being mindful of the stillness of nature and the beautiful sounds that can be found all around us. I was surprised to see how well the children responded to this exercise. They were very respectful. I gave each child a turn to talk about their favorite experiences in nature.

They painted terra cotta pots, played plant identification games and wrote in their journals under a shade tree. We discussed the importance of photosynthesis, cellular respiration and symbiotic relationships. I was impressed that in a class of students ranging from 5 to 12, every student knew what photosynthesis was. Each child gave a great example of a symbiotic relationship. We talked about the parts of a plant and discussed plant families. I taught them about basic medicinal uses for plants and food. We went for a nature scavenger hunt on the nearby college campus, which had a display of plants whose names were inspired by animal names, such as cockscomb, zebra grass and dragon wing begonia.

Day Three. We jumped right into planting the garden. We set the stopwatch for 45 minutes. Each child took turns digging holes, placing plants in the ground, covering them with soil and watering. They were engaged and felt a true sense of accomplishment when the garden was completely planted before the timer went off.

Exhausted from planting, we took a break and made organic berry lemonade with berries from our farm. We also made organic popsicles with juice and berries. The children harvested a basketful of produce from the small school garden that my husband and I installed earlier that spring. They helped wash, prep, slice and shred the vegetables. Then we made rainbow chard rolls filled with chopped vegetables, cheese and organic ranch dressing. Ten out of 12 students cleared their plates.

Day Four. I brought several trays of established seedlings for the children to transplant into painted pots and take home: scallions, black cherry tomatoes, purple peppers, okra, squash, basil and calendula. Each could choose five packets of seeds. They planted one of their seed packets in "mini- greenhouses," recycled plastic clamshell containers and plastic egg cartons filled with soil. We talked about the importance of pollinators and made bird feeders from pine cones. The children cut more vegetables for a healthy snack and enjoyed their homemade popsicles.

The children collected their plants and crafts. We ended the summer camp with a synopsis of what the children learned: why the Earth needs our help, the importance of nature, how we can do our part by reducing our carbon footprint and how to grow our own food. Children around the globe would benefit from these fundamental lessons. It is up to us to plant the seed of Earth stewardship in future generations.

Children Are Like Seedlings

Children and seedlings have similar fundamental needs: sunlight, water, nutrients and fresh air. Without these vital elements, neither could exist. They also both require a solid foundation for their roots. While seedlings rely on their own roots to guide them to be firmly planted into the soil, children rely on their parents, guardians, siblings and mentors to provide them with a loving and supportive environment where they can thrive. They both need room to grow — to spread those roots and reach toward the sky — and need to be nurtured, loved and supported as they mature. As children grow, they slowly integrate experiences in the real world, ultimately enriching their lives and preparing them for the future. They progress from womb to mother's arms to bassinet, followed by crib, small bed, big bed and eventually their own home. Seedlings follow a similar progression. They are started from seed, sprouted in a tiny cell then transplanted into larger pots, hardened off outside and eventually placed into a garden bed or row in a field.

The symbiotic relationship between plants and humans is infinite and cyclical. Our reliance upon plants is a sacred connection, which has been evident and necessary for our survival since the first humans walked the Earth. If children were taught this fundamental lesson at an early age in a way that it would stick with them like the alphabet, they would surely develop a stronger relationship with the natural world and growing up with a basic understanding of how things are connected. From their perspectives, humans need nature and it should not be destroyed. Children's lives would be more magical if they were all given the chance to discover the beauty and wonder of plants, which would surely deepen their connection with the Earth. If we all recognized the importance of caring for the planet, the world would be a better place.

Parents Doing Their Part

I have learned many of my core values from my own wonderful mother, Catherine Moore, who has been teaching in public schools for over 15 years. Her education philosophy is based on the six C's: classroom management, communication, creativity, concern, cooperation and capability. Many of these can be applied to daily life. She helped implement a school garden, which is a fabulous tool for integrating outdoor education with classroom learning. When I asked my mother why she chose teaching, she replied, "I've been guided here, and I plan to teach for all of the little benefits, the children. It is through my grandmother, who nurtured me as she realized my potential, that I speak these words. Children are like flowers. If you nurture them, they will grow and blossom!"

Another amazing mother is my friend, Colleen Smith. She is an herbalist and a homesteader who homeschools her three beautiful and talented girls. Visit her blog at wildstead.wordpress.com.

My dear friend Serene "earthschools" her son Judah and takes him and his baby sister Opal on hikes in the woods several times a day. She is a wonderful example of integrating forest play into daily routine. Her son builds forts instead of playing with electronics. He is also plant savvy. He can recognize wild edibles and medicinal plants. Serene is also a musician, writing songs that offer solutions for environmental concerns.

Kristine Brown is the author and illustrator of the *Herbal Roots* zine, dedicated to teaching children about plants and their medicinal uses. Visit her at herbalrootszine.com.

Rebekah Dawn is an herbalist in my community who home schools her children and started a botanical sanctuary on her land. She creates art inspired by nature.

Teachers, scout leaders, community cultivators, educators, coaches and mentors always deserve acknowledgment. Children thrive on community, positive experiences, workshops, hands-on demonstrations and words of encouragement. Without the guidance and support from family, friends and these community members, children lack a vital component of human

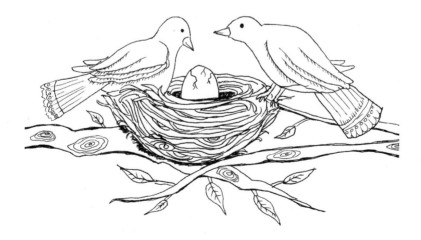

wholeness. Getting children involved in team activities teaches them conflict resolution and symbiotic relationships.

A wonderful way to include children, regardless of their background, is through growing a garden together, whether in their schoolyard, in their neighborhood or in their own backyard. Tending their own garden builds character, teaches responsibility, gives insight into the beauty of nature and fosters their connection with their food sources.

Knowing that one gardening workshop could change the course of a child's life and deepen his or her connection to the world around them is profound. Seeing their eyes light up when finding their very first sun-ripened strawberry and picking it right from the plant brings forth a wave of happiness that cannot be explained.

Those guiding children toward a brighter future make this world a better place. Setting an example is crucial in sculpting them to be compassionate stewards of the Earth.

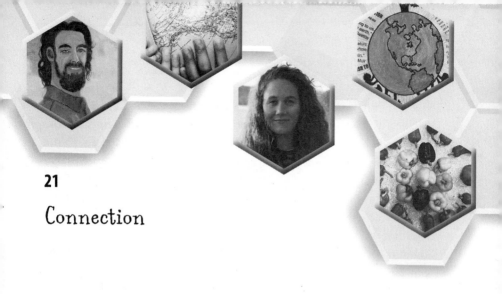

21

Connection

We are all strands in this complex web of life;
moving, twisting, changing directions, gliding parallel ... ever
evolving growing together, growing apart
bonded by the unified strength of the strands themselves ...
mathematically predetermined, designed to thrive with a weave
held together by millions of strands
yet helplessly destroyed by the faintest of winds destined to
intersect
interwoven interconnected interdependent
reliant on one another
remove one strand and the web falls apart ... fiber by fiber
the web disappears

To Live

IN LIFE, there are many paths. In living, there are many choices. In loving, there are many hues. To dream is to awaken to the soft winds echoing through the canyons of time. To be alive is to be in perfect stillness, a spectator to the seasons of change. To be a steward is to hold reverence for all that is symbiotic to the intricate interconnectedness all around us. From the micro-organisms beneath our feet to the symphony orchestra of our feathered friends resting in the treetops and making great migrations just above us ... traveling millions of miles together in unison. The migratory flyways exist over nearly every river in the world. The rivers are the arteries; the streams and tributaries are the life veins of Mother Earth. The trees, her lungs. Our lungs, her breath. This wild beckoning to return to nature exists in each of us who are quiet enough to hear her call. For in the not-so-distant past, we all embraced the wilderness with fearlessness. We were steadfast and strong, wise and intuitive. To stand before an old-growth tree and feel absolutely humbled by its magnificence is to live. To stand before the ocean and bow down knees bent to sand as tears flow freely with every ebb and every flow is to live. To truly hear the ocean waves crash against the dolomite cliffs is to live. To rise above the world in a metal bird and to see the terrain from high in the sky while soaring through the clouds and the warm rays of sun is to live. To climb mountains and stand upon the peak looking out in all directions and seeing the world actually curve at the horizon line is to live. To not take for granted any second of any day is to live. To fill one's heart with pure gratitude for every connection, every interaction, every living breathing organism is to live. To rise with the sun and dream with the moon is to live. To dance around a fire while a drum beat prevails is to live. To look to the skies and see the Northern lights, a meteor shower, billions of stars in the midnight sky is to live. To travel to the wonders of the world is to live. To conceive a child, bringing life-force energy to a being, is to live. And for this embryo to develop and grow in the womb — a miracle we take for granted. To give birth or witness birth is to live. To watch a child grow and learn and discover is to live. To kiss a loved one for the very last time and to witness their very last breath on Earth is to live. To mourn is to live. To be overwhelmed with unwavering sadness is to live. To create is to live. To inspire is to live. To wrap your arms around the love of your life melting into his or her sheer presence is to live. To look another deep, deep in their eyes as if you were looking into a nebula in the cosmos is to live. To feel deep love is to live. To forage wild foods to feed our spirits is to live. To dig our fingertips into the rich dark soils of our gardens is to live. To plant seeds of hope and watch them crack open, rooting deep into the earth while stretching for the sun is to live. To eat from your garden, to feast from the fruits of your own labor, is to thrive. To practice permaculture is to live. To plant trees and gardens is to live. To teach others is to live. To reap what you sow is to live.

To get down close to the earth, breasts pressed against the ground and sinking as far down into the dirt as possible, is to live. To intimately witness the emerging beauty of the plants as they awaken from the damp rich soil that has been lying dormant in the stillness of winter is to live. As the budding shades of green and white make their way through the cold dark layers of earth, the sun's rays shine down so delicately on to their new growth in such a naturally calculated manner; to witness the tiny little microhabitats come to life is to truly live. Knowing that bliss is on the horizon is to live.

In the bitter cold winter, the roots know when to grab hold of the bedrock below, inherently finding the path of least resistance through the decomposing layers of the forest floor. As lateral roots spread and taproots deepen, the stem grows thicker, piercing through the earth's surface to dance its innate dance. The plants have intuition. They know when to sprout, where to set roots, when to flower, when to go to seed and when to go dormant. Their life cycles are in tune with the rhythms of nature, the relationship of the earth to the sun, the soil temperature and the changing seasons. These plants have adapted over thousands of years. But to not be fully aware is to not live, but to slowly wither away inside.

Knowledge is power. The destitution nature feels from the hands of man needs to be healed. It is our intrinsic moral obligation to wake up and care about the world around us. We have ruined the waterways, polluted the air, ripped out the old-growth trees, mined nature to her bare bones and poured salt in her wounds. We must rise up, tear away our selfish skin and hear her plea with every moral fiber of our being. Together, we can return to her. Together, we can begin to slowly reverse the damage we as a race have done. Beyond borders and flags and righteousness lies love. And love begets gratitude. To be grateful and to shed the layers of hatred, fear, bitterness and selfishness is to live. For we cannot live without her.

Rebirth. Rejuvenation. Renewal. Emerging from dormancy and awakening the spirit. Awakening the very essence of our beings is to thrive. Returning to our roots and reclaiming our archaic wisdom is to live. Welcoming the paradigm shift is to live.

> Life's most persistent and urgent question is, what are you doing for others?
>
> — Martin Luther King, Jr.

The world is in dire straits. Philosophers, prophets, educators, healers, scientists, activists, environmentalists, free thinkers, dreamers and the like have been trying to find pragmatic solutions to global epidemics for centuries. In all the searching, love and compassion tend to play a significant role in solutions to hunger and homelessness, poverty, environmental degradation and war, among other severe problems today. World peace will never be possible without love and compassion permeating every cell of our beings. One of my favorite solution-based concepts is *radical compassion*, a term coined by philosopher Khen Lampert, defined as a "specific type of general compassion which includes the inner imperative to change reality in order to alleviate the pain in others." This state of mind, according to Lambert's theory, is universal and stands at the root of the historical cry for social change.

When it comes to matters of the heart, love and compassion are the bringers of joy, the bearers of happiness and the emotions that evoke joyful, visceral responses that make millions smile. Love and compassion have the miraculous ability to heal, to give hope and to actually change the course of one's life. Mindfulness is among the tools needed to truly practice love and compassion in this crazy world. In a world full of love and compassion, trust would grow like wildflowers. Love and compassion were in the core values of some of the most influential peacemakers and religious figures of all time and tend to be recurring themes throughout many religions around the world.

Practice love and compassion daily. Smile at a stranger, offer a hand to someone in need, open doors for others, call a friend to tell them how much they mean to you, practice self-love, go out of your way to do a random act of kindness, pay for the person in line behind you, place coins in toy machines for children, visit the elders in your life, volunteer in your community, be a positive example to others. Positivity, love and compassion send ripples out into the world.

I believe there is a massive disconnect in our modern world between humans and nature. This is most evident in our dissociation from food and our addiction to the conveniences of technologies that are fueled by environmentally destructive practices. The seed-to-table journey is all-encompassing, and it affects every individual around the globe. A day in the life of an average person may very well not include one single moment of contemplation or understanding of nature. But this connection has not been completely lost, as it exists within anyone walking this Earth, whether they recognize it or not. The connection has merely been suppressed in a world so abundant with technological distractions, entertainment, virtual reality and perpetual motion.

Connection is such a vital component of human happiness. Those who possess a deep connection with the natural world seem to have more altruistic connections with other people. In so many ways, it is easy to lose sight of the simple fact that despite our gender, skin color or class or creed differences, we are all human beings functioning together, existing together at this very moment in time, sharing the same cognitive spectrum of emotions of happiness, despair, anger, rage and passion. We are living, breathing organisms with vital organs, skeletal systems, the capability of cerebral processing, we are all covered in skin. We are one and the same yet independently unique. We wander through life, oblivious to the thousands of people we could potentially interact with on just one single day in a calendar year.

Our ability to connect with other human beings is crucial. Positive and negative interactions with others influence our course of action each day. If we are met with negative attitudes from others, chances are we will handle situations in a negative tone. On the other hand, if we are met with pleasantries, most likely we will reciprocate the kindness. Whether it's a friendly smile and brief conversation with the barista in the coffee shop or a pleasant experience with a receptionist in a doctor's office, these positive interactions sculpt our happiness on a daily basis.

It is the small steps in our daily lives that will contribute to a brighter future. The changes Earth stewards want to see in this world are directly rooted in compassion for all life and an ever-evolving deepening in our connection with nature. These changes are possible with a shift in thinking, a unique set of problem-solving skills, a permaculture mindset. Take the basic idea of permaculture and allow the concept as a whole to permeate you in all of your endeavors, keeping in mind how each decision and action affects you, your neighbors, your community, local flora and fauna, the environment, the world and the future.

Each of the problems facing the world today — deforestation, climate change, habitat loss, monoculture, polluted waterways, nonrenewable energy — have been met with a mindset of profit, progress and convenience over concern, compassion and respect. It is desperately time to change this.

Fortunately, people from all walks of life are rising up to form a global transition into a unified vision of sustainability. These people are using everyday actions, small steps, as a way to bring their dreams to fruition. These Earth stewards are planting the way for the next generation; they each leave behind an inspiring legacy for growing, creating and renewing the endless spring of inspiration.

> Never doubt that a small group of thoughtful, committed individuals can change the world. Indeed, it's the only thing that ever has.
>
> — Margaret Mead

Celebrate Earth Day every day!

◉ Eat local, organic and seasonal fruits and vegetables — know your farmer!
◉ Join a CSA farm.

- Shop at your local farmers' market regularly.

- Grow a garden. Try growing and preserving at least 25 percent of your own food. Growing a garden can be super easy and highly rewarding. Container gardening is an option for those who lack space.

- Shop at local mom-and-pop businesses instead of big-box stores.

- Get thrifty: shop at thrift stores. There are so many amazing treasures just waiting for a good home.

- Use cloth bags! Keep a gazillion of them in your trunk so you never have an excuse.

- Walk, bike or use public transportation — or sport a hybrid.

- Ditch the chemicals. Use eco-friendly cleaning supplies.

- There are tons of recipes available at your fingertips for everything from DIY laundry detergent to DIY all-purpose cleaning spray. I use baking soda, vinegar and essential oils to clean. They are cheaper and safer for the environment.

- Make your own body care products. You can make your own lotions, creams, soaps, lip balms and even makeup, using simple and safe ingredients that are better for you and the environment.

- Watch a few documentaries per month. *Awakening the Dreamer, Food, Inc., Hungry for Change* and *Queen of the Sun* are a few good ones to start with.

- Reduce, Reuse and Recycle. These big three have been tried and true for many years.

- Use less water. Instead of buying plastic water bottles, use a stainless steel reusable water bottle.

- Buy tree-free paper for your home and office (www.stepforwardpaper .com).

- Plant a pollinator garden to attract butterflies and honeybees. Landscape with native flowers. Give edible landscaping a try or go with an environmentally responsible company.

- Become a vegetarian or choose to buy meat raised on a biodynamic, earth- and animal-friendly farm.

- Plant a tree each year on your birthday and encourage your friends and family members to do the same.

- Plant fruit trees and perennial fruits in your backyard. Volunteer on a farm or with Slow Foods, the Sierra Club, your local Stream Team or any organization doing good for the community and the environment.

🌀 Spread the information with friends and family members. Start green teams at your office, school or church.

> Small acts, when multiplied by millions of people, can transform the world.
>
> — Howard Zinn

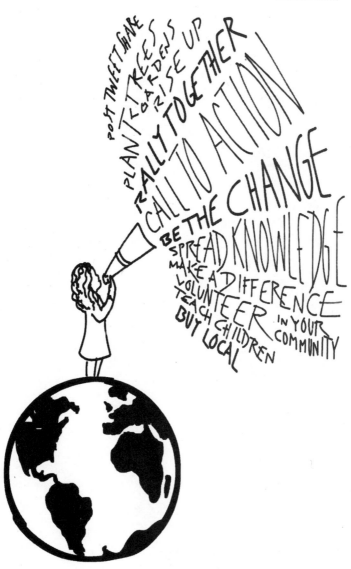

Acknowledgments

WITH PROFOUND GRATITUDE and respect to those who sculpted my professional endeavors and who played a role in being a catalyst for this book to come to fruition...

An enormous, from the bottom of my heart Thank You to my editor and friend, Elena Makansi. This book would not be possible, nor would it be what it is without you, your brilliant insight and the wizardry of words you brought to the book. Thank you for the countless hours you spent on the entirety of this project. It was a privilege and an honor to work so closely with you. Thank you Kristina Blank Makansi for the initial direction and support. I appreciate your dedication to *Grow Create Inspire*.

Thank you Molly Hayden for your encouragement, for the initial edits, for helping me to conceptualize thoughts into words and for teaching me how to use a semi-colon.

Thank you Serene Bardol for your insight, optimism and encouragement of *Grow Create Inspire*.

Thank you to ALL of the amazing women in my life for your authentic friendship and for all the endless inspiration and laughter you bring to my life... especially Serene Bardol, Colleen Smith, Kelley Powers, Molly Hayden, Heather Barth Manley, Brandy McClure Heller, Carolyn Crews, Pooki Lee, Elnora Martinez, Penny Clark and Erin Winkles. My life would not be the same without you.

Thank you Pam Garvey for your insight and words of encouragement and for giving me direction with the initial concept.

Thank you Danette Watt for encouraging me to get my flowery words published. Your support means a great deal to me.

Thank you Bryan Welch, Heidi Hunt, Hannah Aften, Kale Roberts and Robert Riley for welcoming me to the *Mother Earth News* family. Thank you for being a source of inspiration for Earth stewards for so many years. *Mother*

Earth News has brought inspiration and positive change to individuals and communities around the world for decades. Thank you for helping to make the world a better place.

Thank you JB Lester for giving me my beginnings as a writer in *The Healthy Planet* magazine. I am grateful for all that you do for the community.

Thank you to the entire Slow Food St. Louis family!

Thank you Cat Neville, Liz Miller and the entire team at *Feast Magazine* for the opportunity to express my voice as a farmer and forager. It has been an honor to be a part of the *Feast* family.

Thank you Jean Ponzi for the inspiration throughout the years.

Thank you Byron and Beatrice Clemens, Ray Feick, Rich Rodriguez, Jim Scheff and Stephen Brooks for the guidance in my early years.

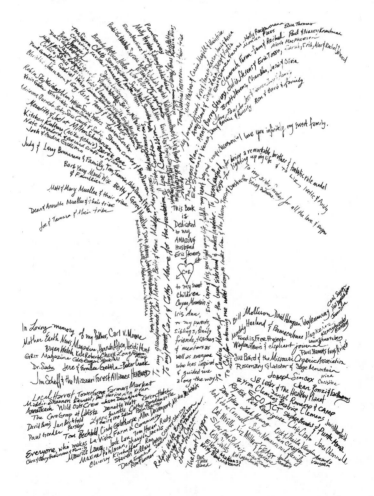

Index

About the Author

C RYSTAL STEVENS is an herbalist, writer, artist, photographer and art teacher, employing multiple platforms to share her passion for inspiring others to care for the environment, to grow gardens, and to live healthy lifestyles. From 2010–2016, Crystal and her husband (along with their two children) managed La Vista Farm, a CSA serving over 150 families on the bluffs of the Mighty Mississippi River. While at La Vista, they farmed 6 acres of diversified vegetables fruits and herbs. During their time at La Vista Farm, Crystal and her husband ran dozens of community outreach programs each year. They hosted field trips and home-school groups, taught gardening and art summer camps for kids, and traveled to inner city schools to present gardening workshops. Additionally, they gave dozens of workshops and presentations on gardening, healthy eating, natural living, medicinal

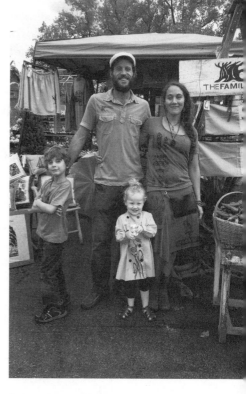

herbs, backyard composting, foraging and other resilient living topics. They are excited to begin their next journey and go where the wild winds blow them.

A Note About the Publisher

NEW SOCIETY PUBLISHERS, is an activist, employee-owned, solutions-oriented publisher focused on publishing books for a world of change. Our books offer tips, tools, and insights from leading experts in sustainable building, homesteading, climate change, environment, conscientious commerce, renewable energy, and more — positive solutions for troubled times.

The interior pages of our bound books are printed on Forest Stewardship Council®-registered acid-free paper that is 100% post-consumer recycled (100% old growth forest-free), processed chlorine-free, and printed with vegetable-based, low-VOC inks, with covers produced using FSC® registered stock. New Society also works to reduce its carbon footprint, and purchases carbon offsets based on an annual audit to ensure a carbon neutral footprint. For further information, or to browse our full list of books and purchase securely, visit our website at: **www.newsociety.com**

New Society Publishers
ENVIRONMENTAL BENEFITS STATEMENT

For every 5,000 books printed, New Society saves the following resources:[1]

30	Trees
2,695	Pounds of Solid Waste
2,965	Gallons of Water
3,867	Kilowatt Hours of Electricity
4,899	Pounds of Greenhouse Gases
12	Pounds of HAPs, VOCs, and AOX Combined
7	Cubic Yards of Landfill Space

[1]Environmental benefits are calculated based on research done by the Environmental Defense Fund and other members of the Paper Task Force who study the environmental impacts of the paper industry.

Certified — (B) Corporation

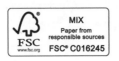

FSC
www.fsc.org
MIX
Paper from responsible sources
FSC® C016245

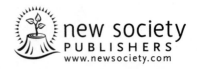

new society
PUBLISHERS
www.newsociety.com